De

and for being a part of our life's journey (through Gem) Dandy
We love you!
Sincerely + God Bless,

The Many Languages & Peaces of God

The Many Languages & Peaces of God

My Journey to Christ...

Through the Twelve Gifts of Grace

Georgianna Penn

Published by Alabaster Book Publishing
North Carolina

The material in this book is not intended as medical advice,
diagnosis or treatment. If you have a medical issue or illness,
consult a qualified physician. Most of the material in this
book is an expression and interpretation of the author's
personal experiences.

For information regarding permission to reproduce
selections from thes book, write to:
Alabaster Book Publishing
P.O.Box 401
Kernersville, NC 27285

Published by Alabaster Books
P.O. Box 401
Kernersville, North Carolina 27285
www.publisheralabaster.biz

Book design by D.L.Shaffer
Cover concept by Georgianna Penn

First Edition

ISBN-13: 978-0-9796866-0-3
ISBN-10: 0-9796866-0-1

Library of Congress Control Number
2007906841

Table of Contents

"The 12 Gifts of Grace"

To my mother
for being my true
source...
And for believing
in and truly
understanding me.

To Vaughanie my
Prayer Warrior
And Guardian Angel

Dedication

To my loving family;
Vaughan, Elaine, Liz,
mom and dad,
who give me wings to fly,
and a safe ground to stand on.

To my dear friends
Tita and Tracy,
my true Earth angels.

To St. Pius the Tenth
Catholic Church
for being my inspiration.

To Karen, Dan and Ethan who brought
me to this little peace of heaven
in the first place.

To my best friend,
Kerry, for
being my rock.

Introduction

Thank you for picking up this book. This is my journey… my faith story.

This book is not necessarily about one religion. It is not necessarily about Christianity. It is; however, about the universal gifts of hope, love and faith.

It is about doing your best everyday, no matter your limitations. It's about finding your own unique wholeness.

I believe God speaks to us in many languages. He gives us many religions, many people and many places in which to share his light and love.

At times, it saddens me that religion can separate so many of us from one another, and that Christianity can be so divided. And, so I've learned when religion builds walls and language fails… it is through this universal gift of love that unites us all together. And no matter our limitations or our differences, we can all find comfort in knowing that God is love.

And, no matter our language or religion, we all have the common goal of love and peace.

My journey has taken me down the path of Christianity, that is my journey.

My prayer for you is to find peace along your journey... to know yourself, know your strengths, know your weaknesses, treat yourself and others with love and respect... and find a way to live life to the fullest, your own unique fullness.

This book is about living life with compassion... and moving through your pain and fear, and learning how to get 'unstuck.' It is about embracing life and living it with grace, dignity and joy.

July 2007

Prologue

This book was journeyed over the past two and a half years. Most of the text in this book originated from a letter; a letter written inviting folks to a very special benefit concert acknowledging mental illness in North Carolina. The letter also reflected my struggles with chronic fatigue syndrome, fibromyalgia and mental stressors. It also reflected my faith journey to the Catholic Church.

The letter was written on January 22, 2007; which, ironically was the same exact date, two years prior, I had first stepped foot into Saint Pius the Tenth Catholic Church… the church to which this book is dedicated.

Unplanned and through many little synchronicities, the letter became a divinely inspired little poetry book. The poetry in this book was also written over the past two and a half years. Each poem has a unique voice, a voice I could finally find and express for my own personal struggles at the time; personal struggles within myself and within the dynamics of certain relationships; and while observing others and their relationships.

Shortly after the letter was written, my friend, Tita, and I discovered each poem could easily be inserted into the letter and therefore; The Many Languages and Peaces of God was born.

The poems became the 12 Gifts of Grace… and in the back of the book you will find a workbook, designed to take through your own unique journey.

I hope you enjoy the pages to come… and find some peace along the way!

July 2007

For I know the plans
I have for you, declares the Lord
Plans to prosper you and not to harm you. Plans to
give you hope and
a future."

Jeremiah 29:11

Hope...
My Faith Story

The journey that has led me this far...

Each and every one of us has a story to tell. I am going to share mine with you. As you may know, I have been managing chronic fatigue syndrome and fibromyalgia for many years now. Along with chronic fevers and flu-like symptoms, chronic fatigue syndrome can be accompanied by a debilitating component of mental fog, brain pain and depression… a temporary loss of healthy cognitive functioning, and a loss of hope.

In turn, this creates a whole new problem, "fear". This fear becomes anxiety and the cycle begins again. At the point I thought was the last flicker of hope, I was taken on a journey with a path leading to a brighter and healthier future, a path leading to hope, love and light... a path leading... to faith.

It began two years ago, January 22nd, 2005, when I woke up in extreme exhaustion, confusion and pain. Overwhelmed by job stressors and an unhealthy relationship, I found myself in the midst of another relapse. The cycle had begun once again. With very little energy to leave my home, and very little mental energy to read or write, I found myself in that agitated frozen state once again. Everyone has a stress response… this was mine, and the worst part is staying stuck in that response, like a skip in a record that can't seem to move forward.

Unable to cognitively figure it out on my own, I was on my hands and knees praying to God to show me where to go and what to do that day. I just needed that jump start, a brief intervention of strength and hope to break the cycle.

I prayed and prayed and finally remembered that Borders Books has Saturday afternoon events that are intellectually and sometimes spiritually stimulating; that would surely snap me out of myself. So, I got into my car and headed towards the book store. But, it began to snow and sleet and Borders was so far away.

Once again, I felt defeated. So, I prayed harder and drove faster…

Prayer - The Soul's Intervention

Prayer
Prayer is reflection
Prayer is faith, Prayer is listening
Prayer is hope, Prayer is thanksgiving
Prayer is sacred, Prayer is communion
Prayer… is the link
The link to love
the link to others
the link to ourselves.
The link… to our God,
"who already knows the needs of
Our hearts, before we even speak them."

G. Penn *November 2005*

this time straight down Elm Street… and I then remembered, "Catholics have church on Saturdays!" Hmmm… As I inched further down Elm Street, my car just seemed to be pulled towards St. Pius the Tenth Catholic Church. I wasn't sure what to do when I got there, I saw the vat of holy water, wondered what to do with it?

I sat in the back of the church so no one would notice my lack of correct hand gestures. And about half way through the sermon, I was offended that the presenter was comparing the recent tsunami to abortion. I got up and attempted to leave. As I approached the door, I thought, "See, those Catholics are so closed minded. How dare they compare one life with another?" Well, little did I know, it was the anniversary of Roe vs. Wade and the speaker was only trying to honor that particular issue. So I stayed.

However, I went to the restroom only to find the stalls were locked. I was having such anxiety that day, my mind filled up once again with fear: "See, Catholics aren't even aloud to use the restroom during mass, they lock the stalls." *In my overwhelmed state, I never imagined some delinquent child had crawled under the doors and locked them as a prank.* I froze once again and remained behind the glass till the end of the mass.

As I contemplated whether I'd ever step foot into that church again, something inside me knew I would. Plus, I had already committed to attend my best friend's baby's baptism that very next week.

I thought I should go since I introduced her and her husband to each other and sang in their wedding. I began to see that everything was connected somehow… and somehow, I was being led.

"I will instruct you and teach you in the way you should go; I will counsel you and watch over you." Psalm 32:8 (New International Version)

So, Feb. 5th, 2005 was the day. Ethan Goodin was to begin his life in the light of Christ. Throughout the mass, I was truly moved, completely absorbed in the beautiful ceremony that bonded this family together. Ethan was the funniest and cutest of all, of course. And little did I know, this was the intervention and "jumpstart" my soul so desperately needed.

At the end of the ceremony, the deacon and priest invited everyone up for their flu shot. I was confused. They then proceeded to explain the story of *St. Blaise,* patron saint for the healing of throats… and gave each one of us a throat blessing with tall beautiful crossed candles. I was afraid to go up, but my friends took me by the hand and led me up front for a healing. It was the most magical moment I had ever experienced.

Thc next day I was light and happy and the aches and pains were gone and my chronic sore throat was healed, at least temporarily. I had just experienced my first Catholic ritual. Awesome! I went to church again that Sunday. I began to go every week, and even on weekdays in the afternoons, usually when I felt the worst.

On the weekends I had to attend all three ceremonies to be able to fully hear and download the sermon. I had never in my life, anywhere in the country, experienced such a spirit filled place… and they were smart and loving too, what a great combination! I learned so much, mostly spiritual truths I already knew, but could never find the words for or fully express myself. I began to write poetry and sketch little inspirations everyday after mass… it was a true healing! I was truly inspired and had found a way to express that inspiration.

Sometimes art, music and poetry can reach parts of our souls that basic language could never reach. That is what the sermons at St. Pius have done for me. And that kind of creative expression, whether created or endured, acts as sort of a bridge. A bridge, between joy… and pain.

ART

The Soul's Expression

"Paint 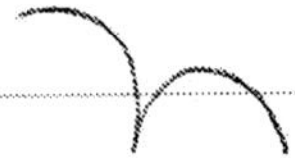

your soul

to PEACE..."

"Art is the bridge between

Joy 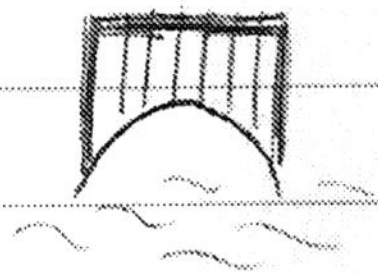

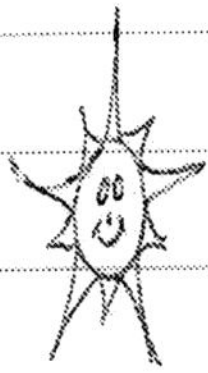 & Pain...

Sunshine... & Rain"

"ART" – The Bridge Between Joy and Pain

I believe God speaks to us in many languages.
And art is one of those languages in which
He shares his light and love.
It is that little reminder of God's love and
salvation here on Earth and in the big picture.

I began sketching about a year ago to soothe
the pain and fatigue of fibromyalgia
and chronic fatigue syndrome.

Unable to enjoy aerobics and dance on a
consistent basis as a therapeutic outlet, I became
more frustrated and fatigued.

Discovering art as a healing outlet was a life
saver.

Sketching and drawing shifts the brain
Away from the stress of pain and fatigue into a
peaceful steady flow.

It calms the mind, soothes the soul and frees my emotions; therefore, re-setting the pain signal and locking in a steady calm.

And being able to reach that state of peace here on earth… gives me hope and faith in the bigger picture.

That 'peace'… is the peace of God...
It is a mere snapshot and little reminder of the peace that is to come through our Salvation.

I believe God speaks to us in many languages… through art, music, the work that we do, the many gifts and talents and even challenges that are bestowed upon us.

Our souls are constantly striving to be closer to God… and even though we may not always 'feel' him or see him… he is always there, waiting to be reached, waiting to be shared.

For God is that bridge between joy and pain.

G. Penn May 2006

Hope

The Soul's CPR

I attended mass four times a week for many months. It was so nice to hear what I believe to be true in a way I could understand and voice myself. The sermons were brilliant. I was so thankful to be open to this place. See, I believe God is always there waiting to be reached, we just can't always feel him or see him… but, when we do, it is to be cherished. Those moments are beautiful and magical. And so I thank you St. Pius.

Many, many months of clarity, focus and happiness went by… I hadn't been that healthy in five years!

However, more stressors came my way, and I crashed once again. However, this time I had a new armor, "hope." I had experienced six months of blissful hope… and even though I was angry I had fallen again, looking back, I learned the true meaning of hope. I was given the gift of "hope".

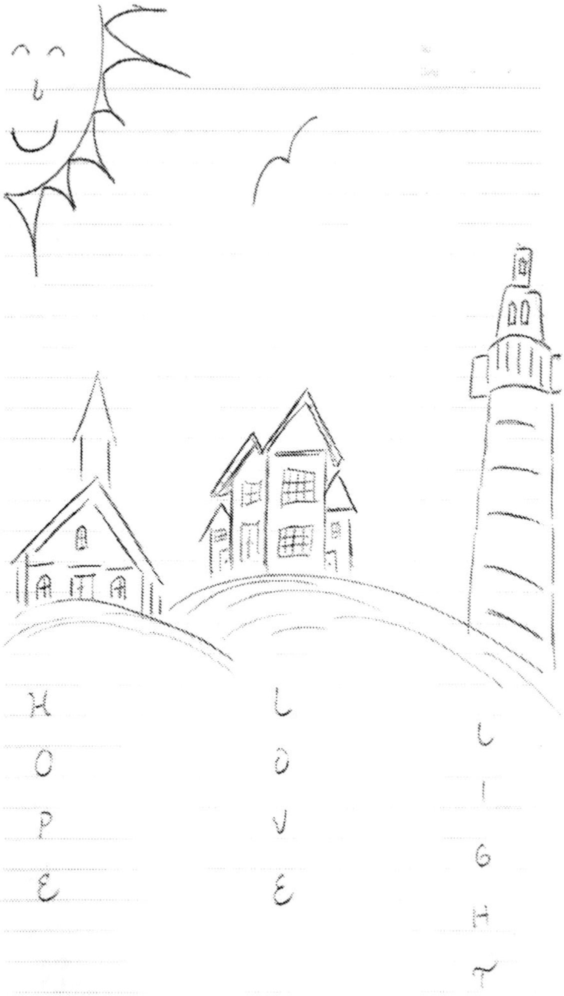

mar. 2006 G. Penn

Hope

Sometimes, the soul begins
to heal long before the
body and mind
even know they are ready.
We go places
we never imagined we would go…
And we are moved in ways
we never imagined we
could be moved…
The Soul knows its journey… long before it's
begun. However, when life gets overwhelming,
It's easy to be blinded by its
stressors and fears,
And miss all of Gods beautiful blessings
along the way.
And sometimes, those fears can
turn into years
in darkness.
However, all we ever really need
is a little, tiny, miniature
ray of hope,
and we are on our way.
A tiny sign that clearly reveals
The pathway before us
As one of hope,
love and light.
May your soul be grounded always
in Hope, Love and Light.

G. Penn July – Dec. 2005

The 12 Gifts Continued

"Old habits can't be thrown out the upstairs window.
They have to be coaxed down the stairs
one step at a time." Mark Twain

Love Your Shadow

That summer, I began the Catholic catechumen program, RCIA. Everyone encouraged me to join. I wasn't sure I wanted to actually become "Catholic"... for I was just truly learning about love and hope. I wrote more poetry, attended church, met with a few leaders in the church I call my spiritual guides... they call them "sponsors". I was in RCIA and wanted to finish. There was so much to learn, but I was so overwhelmed with life's stressors, I continued to have many more relapses. However, I was learning valuable lessons in hope, love and faith.

I wanted to finish the program just in case one day I may want to become Catholic. I felt undue pressure as Easter approached and sort of sabotaged myself from joining the church that particular year. I kept finding reasons why I wasn't ready. I wanted to be fully unassociated with my unhealthy relationship before participating in the sacraments. I also had very little discipline in life. Constantly battling chronic fatigue and pain can keep you stuck in a perpetual victim mode.

I began to dislike all those parts of myself. I pretended like they didn't exist. And so therefore, they screamed louder to be heard and continued to bring me down. So, once again I reached out to one of my spiritual guides seeking the never ending hope he usually extends. Only to find this time, he offered not hope, but a challenge. He said, "Georgianna, you have to be whole before you can become holy." Well, needless to say, I was devastated by this comment. I once again began running in circles trying to find the missing pieces of my fragmented self. I looked for myself everywhere else but myself. I wanted to have the same schedule and amount of energy as others. I wanted to learn things cognitively, not just by feel. But, I only came to find me where ever I looked. And if I kept trying not to be me, I just had more relapses. I couldn't even be around my loving family, their natural traits of anxiety and stress only triggered more pain and fatigue in me. I was in a terrible cycle and had put myself under the utmost microscope.

When we try and untangle the webs of our past… remember, don't abandon those parts of yourself. For they need love too.

Love Your Shadow

When we try and untangle
the webs of our past,

Remember...
don't abandon those parts of yourself.
Because they will only come back
even bigger.

Instead...
acknowledge them and accept them.

For they need love too.

And one day... maybe... just maybe, they won't
scream so loud to be heard.

And they will no longer need to be
in the driver's seat of your life.

G.Penn *Sept. 2006*

"If I speak in human and angelic tongues, but do not have love, I am a resounding gong… or a clashing cymbal."

1 Corinthians 13:1 (NAB)

It's Only Love That Heals

Luckily, I learned those family *reactions* are just family dynamics, not family problems. I learned our family and friends are our biggest assets. I also learned that no matter what, you are who you are. Our strengths are our weaknesses, and our weaknesses our strengths. So, I guess what I am saying is honor who you are and make the best of who you are. There will always be limitations, so focus on the strengths... and if you cannot do it on your own, find others who will help you reach your best self. That is what St. Pius, my friends and amazing family have done for me.

I now believe we have our *own unique* wholeness to reach no matter our limitations. I live with this truth everyday. I believe we should reward ourselves and others for the tiniest of accomplishments… and when we fall, know that it is ok to get back up and start over again and again and again.

"For a just man falleth seven times, and riseth up again."

Proverbs 24:16 (KJV)

However, sometimes we are unable to get back up on our own, we need others to help guide us back to ourselves and walk with us along the path towards healthier daily living and break the cycle, even if it's just for a day.

It's Only Love That Heals

Time is a healer
But not so much without love.

Hospitals, doctors, therapists,
They're all great healers,
But very little can 'stick'
Without Love.

Hard work, self discipline
And structure… these
All keep us balanced,
But without Love,

There's just not enough
Fuel to power
These self healers.
The soul's journey is meant to be
Done alone,
But not completely alone.
No one can hold our hand
And do it for us…
But they can take us by the hand
And walk with us in Love.

G.Penn Summer 2006

"Touched by Grace"

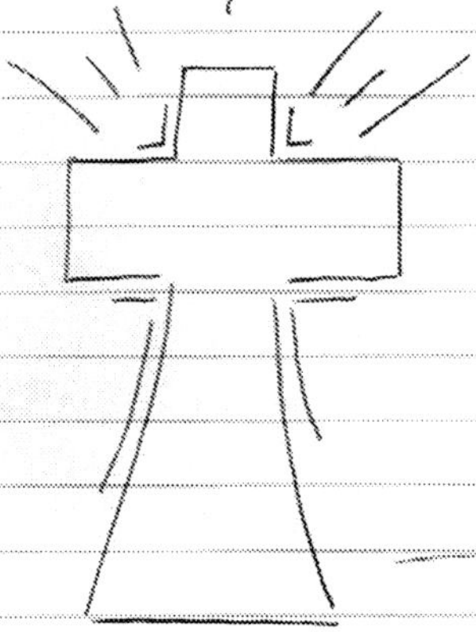

at

Saint Pius the Tenth

by:
Georgianna Penn

I know now that I learn by "feel" not so much by intellect. That's a strength, but also a weakness. I can go an entire month and not plan one day… just wake up and go where I think I should go for the day. I thought for so long that was a terrible way to be. But the more I pushed away that trait, the bigger it got. I am also extremely emotional, so I crave the linear side of life. It doesn't come as natural, but when I distract my emotions with concrete structure, it gives me balance. And so I find that at St. Pius I not only feel God, but the concrete structure and beliefs of the church ground me as well. *Sometimes, when the mass is too emotionally intense for me to attend, on those days, I just remain behind the glass.*

I am not sure when or if I will ever become Catholic, but I do know when I get off course and the fog is too thick to decipher the way, St. Pius is the light to which I am drawn over and over again. And so I ask for your prayers of clarity and peace regarding my spiritual journey towards the Catholic faith.

Once again, I beleive God speaks to us in many languages, he gives us many people, many places and many religions in which to share his light and love.

Each Other - Our Closest Access

When I first began attending St. Pius, a Catholic friend of mine so curtly reminded me that in the Catholic faith, we are not encouraged to follow one priest or parish. We are encouraged to worship no matter who the Priest is, no matter who the people are. When you join the Catholic Church, you're joining the Catholic Church Universal. Well, I tried really hard not to let that comment discourage me since it had been so many years since I'd been inspired in such a way as I have been at St. Pius.

See, all of my life, I have always experienced God through other people… They are like that little jumpstart we all need at times. And so, I believe our closest access to God is through other people, through each other.

Other people are our closest access to God…

They serve as guides along the way. They take us by the hand, heart and mind and inspire us or challenge us. They help us learn who we are… and who we are not. Sometimes, they even pick us up and carry us. And sometimes, they challenge us to come out of the dark and face those parts of ourselves that need the most love and rehabilitation.

And since God is in each of us… "we" are our closest access to him. Or at least initially. However, we are not to become totally co-dependent on each other and diffuse our connection with him. We are to try and come to our relationships with our own God-like center. But, when we have completely gone astray and have no strength of our own, God does give us others to help jumpstart his existence in us once again.

"God transcends all creatures. We must therefore continually purify our language of everything in it that is limited, image-bound or imperfect, if we are not to confuse our image of God – "the inexpressible, the incomprehensible, the invisible, the ungraspable" – with our human representations." Catholic Catechism. See Source Notes.

"Since our knowledge of God is limited, our LANGUAGE about him is equally so. We can name God only by taking his creatures as our starting point and in accordance with our human ways of knowing and thinking" Catholic Catechism. See Source Notes.

On Family & Friends

I believe our friends and family, and other special people who come into our life are like little angels… little messengers of hope, love and light. They are sent here to teach us exactly what we need to learn at that exact time. Whether to inspire us or challenge us, we are to honor this gift; this gift of friends, this gift of family, this gift… of each other.

On Baptism

Besides honoring one another through our basic daily living, in the Christian faith, there are actual spiritual rituals or "sacraments" that represent and affirm this bond with others. In the Catholic faith, seven sacraments are recognized, whereas in the Protestant faith, only two or three are typically recognized.

Through the sacrament of Baptism, we are committing to our family of origin, to take care of each other with Christ in the center of all of our interactions… to do our best to love our family.

On Communion, Community and Church

Through the sacrament of Communion, we are committing to sharing the gift of Christ with our community… *friends, family and church.* To do our best to respectfully love and honor one another. Once we are blessed with this sacrament, we are then meant to go out into the world and share it with others.

And so once again, it is through each other that we are given the gift of community, the gift of church. Without each other, there would be no community… no body of Christ.

On Religion & Spirituality

And so, whether you attend an actual church or just bond with friends and family spiritually, God gives us each other to help us grow in his light and love, and help one another reach the ultimate goal… the ultimate goal of being closer to him and him to us. The ultimate goal of Salvation.

Someone recently said to me... *when I told them of my journey to the Catholic faith,* they said with such conviction: "remember Georgianna, it is religion that separates people." Well, needless to say, I was instantly filled up with fear… thinking of going back to those days of isolation, when I was perfectly content going to church in my own living room every Sunday morning, with channel 4 playing in the background, not having to deal with any one religion or church, when I realized…

It's not religion that separates people… it's people who separate people. It's the disrespect and manipulation of religion or anything else, in any human interaction that separates us.

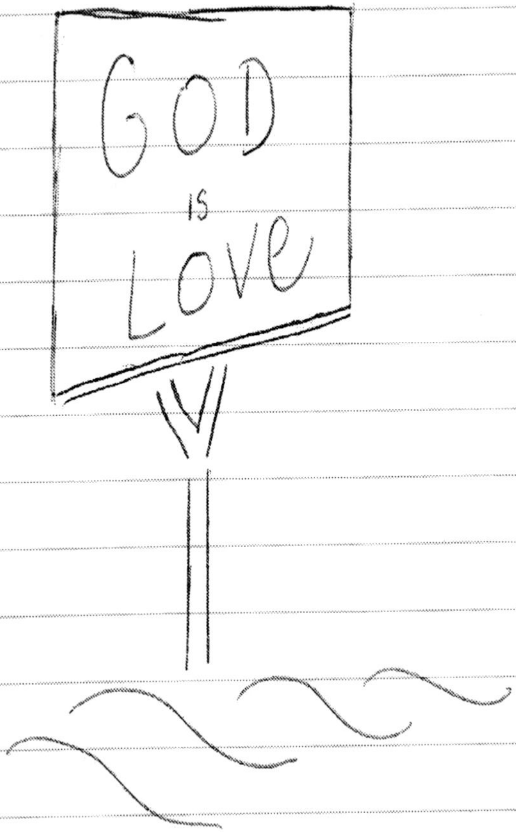
GOD
IS
LOVE

And so I thank God for this realization, and continue my journey towards the Catholic faith.

I find that religion is like a blueprint or guideline designed to keep us on track towards being our best selves… for ourselves, for each other and for God.

And so I guess what I am trying to say is honor one another.

We are not perfect, we are not God. However, we are all made in the image of God. And so we are meant to honor this gift; this gift… of each other.

Compassion

Compassion

I will not take on your pain,
For it is yours, and yours alone.
For how can you truly heal if I have taken it
from you.
For I am compassion,
Not empathy.
I will not shower you with
self pity and sorrow,
For I am compassion, not sympathy.
I will love you
with all my heart,
But I will not give it to you to keep.
For I am compassion, not your martyr.
For how can I love you
if I have given it
away.
I will listen to you and support you
I will not hinder you, nor enable you.
For I am compassion,
not co-dependence.
I will seek to understand you,
and if I am unable
to relate…
I will still armor you
with strength and love,
Because I am compassion,
And it is compassion
that carries us through.

G. Penn Feb. 23, 2006

Now, after two years, I have been struggling with how I can give back to others in similar situations. I still at times find myself in that survival/victim mode... and wonder how in the world could I possibly help someone else. But once again, the answer came to me through my family, friends and St. Pius.

The start was as simple as my dear friend, Tita, showing me a club that would be a great place to host a concert for my sister. When I approached my sister, she suggested we organize a concert for a charity. As if cued from above, we both decided instantly, that a mental health organization was to be the recipient of this idea.

My family and I share the same passion for helping others and wanted to give back to something related to the church and the community. So, I thought of my new RCIA friend, Jodi Lorenzo-Schibley, Executive Director of Sanctuary House.

When I learned of the programming and mission at Sanctuary House, I knew it was the perfect match. I was amazed to find a place that actually focused on strengths and not limitations, a place to do things with others, and not just sit and talk about one's problems. Sanctuary House seemed to be a place that teaches the very essence of living life to the fullest, no matter our limitations.

So, I contacted Jodi and told her of the show and asked if she would be interested in setting up a booth and donation jar at our show.

Well, the very next week, I picked up Jodi and drove her to the music venue. As soon as we arrived, the promoter had some news to share with us… they were closing their doors as of December 31, 2006 and the show was to be cancelled.

Wow! We had three bands booked to play and a charity to raise money for… and no place to call home. Luckily, we presented the idea to the Sanctuary House board and had an amazing response. Sanctuary House was to take on the show as a full blown benefit concert!!

From that point on, Sanctuary House worked so hard on making this an event to remember. The marketing, the invitations, the new venue we had to find… it all just fell into place… It was an unbelievable honor teaming up with such amazing people.

Jodi Lorenzo-Schibley is truly a gift to the mental health community. Her interpersonal counseling and communication skills surpass any amount of education… she is truly gifted beyond her years. And, along with her board, Jodi is the lifeline of Sanctuary House of Greensboro.

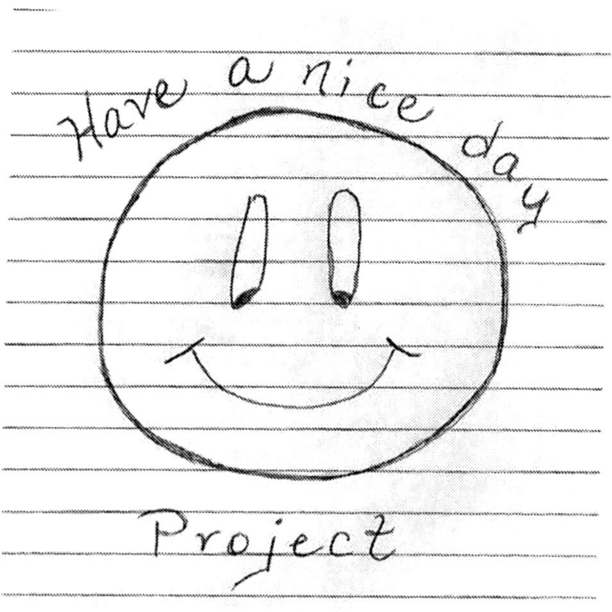

When organizing my family's band and Vaughan for the show, I wanted to include someone else… someone who has been a support for me at this church and someone whose music has been waiting patiently to be heard. That someone is Tracy Welliver. His beautiful and peaceful soul was sort of that final peace this show needed. I thoroughly enjoyed sharing this evening with Tracy and his wife and the very special Wofford family, who performed with him. That night, Feb. 10th, 2007, was a tremendous success! Sanctuary House and its many supporters raised over $50,000… gained new followers and new friends. The members shared their stories and Sanctuary House worked so hard, as if they were planning for a night at the Grammy's!

Using your talents and gifts to help others is truly like coming full circle. Using those gifts with friends and family completes that circle. It was so exciting bringing together old and new friends for this cause. Thank you Sanctuary House for taking us on. See, I believe compassion is the true essence of Christianity...

"When we use our unique gifts to help others, we are fulfilling our mission as a Christian."

Sue Brusnahan

And the Greatest of These

That same great spiritual guide whom I spoke of earlier, also once said...

"When language fails, there's always the universal gift of love, given to us through art, music, other people, family and friends."

In the Catholic faith, there are two types of grace; actual grace and Sanctified grace. Actual grace is anything from art, music, a beautiful sunset or an inspiring person or place. Sanctified grace is the seven Christian sacraments.

So according to the Catholic faith, I have experienced God most of my life through actual grace. God has blessed me with so many of these amazing graces… my heart is filled with gratitude for that. See, God is always, always there, so close, waiting to be reached. Waiting there patiently, with the Greatest gift of all…

Love

Love

It is love
that lights the way,
love that unites
us all together.

It's love
that transcends fear.
And love, that endures us forever.

May your soul
be grounded in love,
And love will light your way.
And remember, love with all
your heart and your
mind.

For it is love that
heals all wounds
And Love…
That brings us home.

G. Penn *Nov. 2005*

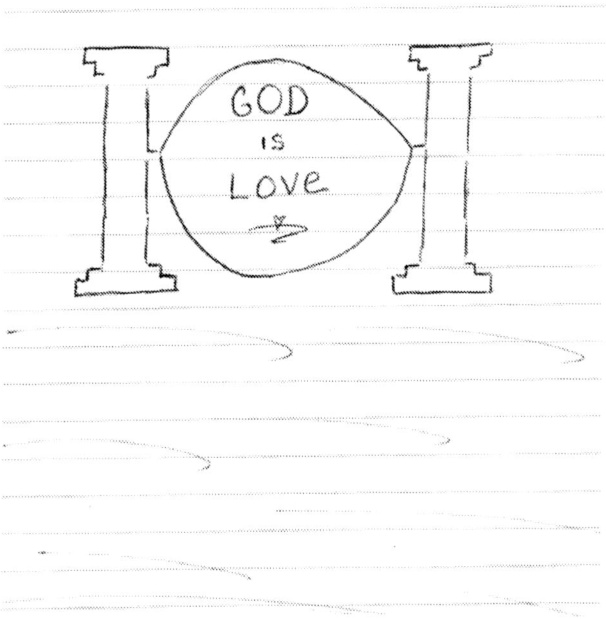
GOD
IS
LOVE

And so I've learned, when we don't speak the same language or process life in the same way, or when mental stressors impede our language… it is through this universal language of love, through very special people like you and special places like Sanctuary House, that brings us hope. And that hope grounded in love, gives us faith.

And so I am not sure where I will go from here, but I do have faith that the same great force that has led me this far, will not lead me astray in the future. I now have faith. I've been given the gift of *faith.*

Faith

Faith

Faith is patience,
Waiting and trusting in
God's timing.

Faith is action... Taking steps when there
are seemingly no steps to take.

Faith is knowing... Knowing that
with every step we take
Our faith and will
only grow stronger.

Faith… is letting go.
When our own attempts only leave us stuck
or running in circles,
Faith is letting go.

Not giving up, but giving it all up to him.

Faith…
Faith is peace.
That confident assurance
that he is there with us
Guiding us and protecting us
As we step out patiently…in faith.

G. Penn *July '06*

Gratitude

I hope you enjoy my poems and essays in the pages to come. And once again, I thank God, my friends and family and all the amazing graces along the way for being that shining light that leads me, guides me and grounds me. It is my hope to share that hope with others, and know that when the fog gets too thick to decipher the way, have faith… never let go of the tiniest flicker of hope and fill your hearts always with gratitude and you are on your way.

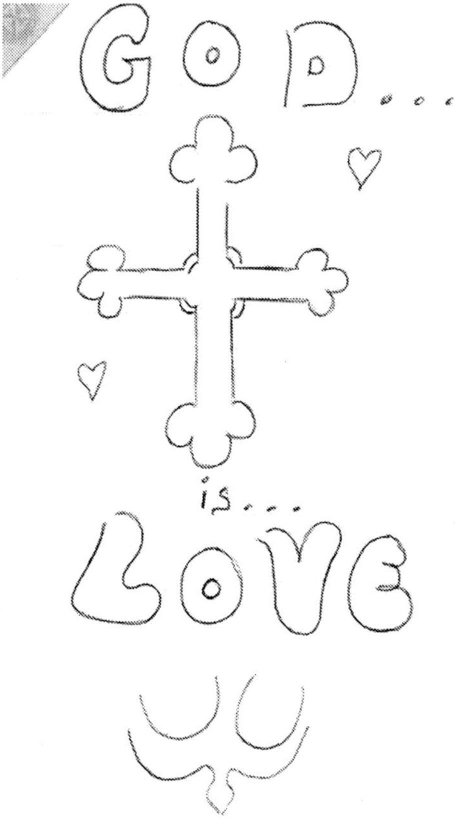
GOD...
is...
LOVE

Gratitude

Open your heart and mind
to God's beauty
all around you.

See the Lord
in everything you do.

And fill your thoughts and soul
everyday with gratitude.

For if we are
filled with gratitude
Then there is very little room
for that which drains us.

For it is gratitude
that strengthens us
beyond pain and fear.

And gratitude is the one true
path towards love…
and peace.

G. Penn July 2006

Courage

The active component
of hope, love & faith.

I was praying for the courage I did not have and could not have found it on my own. I thought, if they can do it, so can I. Thank you Sanctuary House, Jodi, and especially its members for inspiring me towards courage.

I have now left my job of seven years and my relationship of five years.

I am now able to take the steps needed towards my own unique wholeness. I have been given the gift of courage. Thank you, courage.

When sharing my rough drafts with one of my favorite college professors, she summarized this section of my book with the following quote:

"The enemies of courage are fear and depression, especially as we find ourselves faced with our own limitations. When we learn to accept, to live with and to embrace our limitations; though fractured we are… God makes us whole."

Well, this amazingly true quote summed up this section perfectly. And so I am referring to it as the introduction to courage.

Time and time again, over the past seven years, I would find myself 'stuck' in those negative effects of life. Stuck in fear, stuck in pain, stuck in depression… stuck in unhealthy relationships and situations, with no end in sight. And so, I've learned that it's not fear, depression or illness that are the enemies; it's the 'staying stuck' that's the enemy. The loss of hope, the unmanaged limitations, the unmanaged fear, pain and depression.

So, this next section describes some of those negative effects of life and how to attempt to manage them, *or at least acknowledge and recognize them.* And move through them. And to some extent, know that these adversities are gifts too... and that they help us to grow and learn.

I truly believe I could not have known courage without adversity.

You can't know courage,
Really know courage
if you haven't known fear,
intimately.

On Fear

Has anyone ever tried to fill you with their fear? So much, that they won't stop until you feel their pain. And if you don't give in, they just keep pushing their fear further and further at your soul. Well, it's their fear, not yours. That should give us comfort that we don't have to go down with their sinking ship. But, when it's someone on which you are dependent... a parent, sibling, boss, spouse, whatever, it makes it so much harder.

And if you already have a 'fear disorder'... *a chronic illness, depression, anxiety,* or you have so much stress with your own life, it's like fuel on the fire; like hot daggers stabbing your soul.

Find some peace. You are not a victim, it's just the dynamics at that particular moment. Have the wisdom to know if it's your fear, or the fears and issues of someone else. Don't blame others, just try to manage your thoughts and feelings and manage how much time, energy and strength you give to others' fears and issues.

"Fear"

Hi, my name is fear.
I come in many shapes
And sizes…And disguises too.

If I come to your door,
I may try and convince you to let me in,
I may even ask you to feed me
And be my friend.

I am constantly hungry and lonely too,
And cannot exist without
Strength from you.

I am designed to alert you to danger
And motivate you to safety.
So if I knock,
Acknowledge me…
And I will politely go away.

But if you let me in, I am here to stay.
And if you feed me,
I will constantly need more
Because I am fear,
Truly empty
At the core.

I have no strength of my own,
And once I am your reality…
Well, then… I've found myself
A permanent home.

So keep me at bay and save your soul,
Because I am fear
a true black hole.

G. Penn *2006*

On Depression

Depression isn't always sadness or gloom, sometimes it's just glue; brain freeze and neuro-fatigue. Sometimes it's a response, a stress response to so much mental pressure others put on us or we put on ourselves.

Sometimes it's from staying too long in a very stressful or dysfunctional relationship. Sometimes it's from abusive or invasive bullying from others. Sometimes it's from not using our gifts, and sometimes it can come from unfortunate life circumstances like change, loss, illness, death or injury.

Dear Readers,

Hello, my name is depression. You may have heard of me, you may have even seen me. Maybe I'm that person down the street or that girl next door. Or, maybe I'm even closer to you than you think.

Well, Webster's knows me. Webster refers to me as "an area lower than the surrounding surface; sadness and gloom; emotional dejection and withdrawal greater than that warranted by any objective reason."

Well, I know me too, better than Webster. Better than some far off fancy definition that describes someone else, and barely scratches the surface of who I really am.

I present myself in many different ways… many symptoms, many manifestations. I am triggered by many different triggers, manifesting myself uniquely in each suffering victim.

The fog, the inability to find words and communicate, the frustration… is all like looking through a murky windshield without the strength or clarity to turn on the wipers. And not only are you unable to turn on the windshield wipers, but you can't find them... and you can't find them because you have forgotten where they are.

See, depression is like temporary brain damage, not structurally, but cognitively. Sometimes, you find yourself running in circles, trying to escape the mental fog and pain. And, sometimes, you just find yourself frozen in so much mental and physical exhaustion, you're unable to find the desire and strength to reach out and escape yourself. When you've lost the ability to reach out… you are in pretty deep.

Whatever your pain, emotional sadness and fear, or just frozen neuro-fatigue, depression can be triggered by so many triggers. And, it effects everyone, the young, the old, the sick, the healthy, the very poor, and the very wealthy.

No matter your symptoms, no matter who you are… never stop reaching out. Never, ever stop reaching out. Have patience, be kind to yourself and have faith. Eventually, you will find someone to take you by the hand… if not hold your hand, and walk with you out of the fog.

The answers to depression do not lie in this essay. This is merely my attempt to share a small glimmer of hope. Know yourself. Be kind to yourself and others. Rest when you need rest. Be active when you need to be active.

According to the Barnes & Noble Concise Medical Dictionary, there are two types of depression… neurotic and psychotic. Neuro meaning of the central nervous system. Psychotic meaning of the mind. Neurotic depression is also called "reactive depression", it occurs as a reaction to stress. Psychotic depression is called "endogenous depression", it occurs spontaneously in the mind.

Reactive depression is like any other stress response, if already stressed, reactive depression can occur as quickly as an asthma attack… the brain freeze can feel like the most stuck, cognitive glue you could ever imagine.

Reactive depression is the only type I am able to speak of. The brain wants to shift, but can't. Everyone is different, so get to know yourself, and manage your energy. You will eventually figure out how to shift. This type of depression feels very physical… it is of the central nervous system, so the symptoms are physical. The agitation, the stuck brain… feels like the worst ADD moment that just can't seem to pass.

Please contact your licensed health care provider if you feel you are experiencing depression… or any support groups in your area. If you are looking for a community to help you live your life more fully, try your church community or contact a Clubhouse Model psychiatric rehabilitation center in your area.

Depression can be triggered by a physical illness, life changes, job loss, unhealthy relationship dynamics with loved ones or at work… poor diet, lack of sleep and any other type of stress you could possibly imagine.

The brain is very complex. If you could image how complex outer space is and how very little we know about it, then you've imagined the human brain.

Do your best everyday… if you can no longer focus long enough to play chess, play checkers. The brain loves a sense of accomplishment, even if it's the tiniest of accomplishment!

Please see my workbook for some ideas on brain stimulation. Please note: this essay only provides hope and coping ideas… please see a licensed health care provider if you are experiencing depression. If your loved one is too overwhelmed to reach out, consider contacting someone for professional help. Be patient and listen.

On Overreaction

Just a moment ago, I reminded you to never stop reaching out. However, chronic overwhelmed overreaction can keep us 'stuck' too… in a manic, circle-talk, rambling and exhausting cycle. So, balance is key. And try to manage all of your traits, so they don't keep you 'stuck' running in circles… and sabotaging your *full-life* you deserve to live.

Journal Entry on Overreaction
October 22, 2005

When you're overwhelmed with your day, your schedule, your life, your bills, your relationship, etc… and you reach out in such desperation to someone; and you're overreacting with such anxiety, using lots of words, but saying nothing… *at least not anything that makes sense*, you can expect them to either not understand you or misunderstand you. And, when you keep pushing and pushing, well, they have to answer you, especially, if you are giving them all your power, putting all your worries and concerns in their hands; then, they **will** take control. And sometimes, you may not like what they say or do in response to your overreaction. But, you've just reached out in such desperation, that the person you reached out to is overreacting too… setting up a whole chain reaction of overreactions. Like putting out fires over and over and over again. So, before your primary language becomes one of permanent overreaction, know yourself. Manage your worries and process them somewhat before reaching out. Or, you may waste lots of time and energy if you allow 'overreaction' to become your primary language.

Note: If this paragraph made you feel like overreacting… then, you get the picture!

More traits...

that keep us stuck in exhausting patterns.

Feel free to insert any word in place of "artist"... for example: *doctor, actor, writer, professional athlete, "the boss", entrepreneur, inventor, "poor me" or victim. I'm sure we all know someone or some part of our own personality that at times fits some portion of this poem. Have fun! And Please note: When reading aloud, please use humor.*

The Poor Me Starving Artist

I am completely unplugged from society, for I live in my own world, a world of my perceptions and my reality.
I am so full of myself, for no one else exists. I have no respect for others' feelings, for I am only concerned with how they effect me.
I so desperately need drama to create my world that I bring chaos to every interaction… contaminating all in my path with my own fears and realities.
I'm all enmeshed and have no thoughts of my own and will take over your world if you let me… for I am starving and an artist and need you to survive.
Like a host in the human body, moving from part to part, sucking all life… making it my own… my song, my dance, my world, not yours.
I know it all, for I am a prophet… for I am an artist.
I have no social grace… for I see right through you and will tell you exactly what I see with little or no concern for your destiny.
I am so desperate to be "right", that I make others sick or crazy just from my fight.
For I am starving… and always will be if I remain in this prison. This prison… of me, me, me.

G. Penn April 6th, 2007

The Spoiled Rotten Brat

She will take the clothes right off your back…
She likes yours better,
And that's that.

She will whine and complain,
Until you, go insane.
And then blame you for being
The one… who's crazy.

She's the only one
In the world.
And constantly needs
More, more, more.

She demands your attention
With her 'spoiled rotten'
Pleas.

And will take your soul,
And still…
Not… be pleased.

Georgianna Penn May 18th, 2007

Addiction

Don't put your addiction on me.
Addiction destroys.
It destroys the mind, body and soul.
It eats away our very existence
Like a festering cancer.
So, don't put your addiction on me.
It destroys entire family dynamics.
So, don't put your addiction on me.
It steals.
It lies.
It justifies.
It atrophies the very functioning
Of the human body and mind.
So, don't put your addiction on me.

No matter how big or how small,
Don't put your addiction on me.
For if you do, you may as well have
Given me a life sentence or a
Deadly disease.
So, don't put your addiction on me.

G.Penn July 2007

The Narcicist

If you're not showing me attention,
Well, then, I guess you don't like me.
My problems are so much bigger
Than yours, can't you see?
If I'm not the center
Of your party,
Well, then, I am
Not able to attend.
And, if you're not sharing
Your deepest darkest secrets
with me,
Well, then, I guess
I'm not your friend.
I have no concern
For your journey or pace,
For I am the only one in this place.
I'm a master manipulator...
I will tell you what to do
And when and how to do it,
In a way that best suites me.
For, I cannot handle rejection,
Because it is all
About me,
Can't you see?

G.Penn July 2007

Sometimes getting stuck in 'me-mode' can take us over, like a festering disease. Once you are heading down this destructive path, there's no end in sight. Your cup can never be filled because of the destructive and erosive patterns. But, there is always a chance to recognize when your 'self' is taking over. There are many exit ramps to take, you do not have to get so far down this path that you can't turn back. Recognizing what and who triggers this self-ishness is key. Just being *aware* is the first step to managing any unhealthy behavior pattern.

On Living With Our Limitations

Imagine you are on a trip and you know your vehicle. You know it burns oil more quickly than your previous cars. And, if you're taking a long trip and you have not recently serviced your car, then you will need to be extra prepared in order to maintain your car's oil challenge. You will need to keep a stock of oil in your trunk or car. You will need to check your oil frequently throughout your trip. You'll need a funnel and some paper towels. You just need to be prepared, no matter your cars' limitations.

You will also need a set of boundaries. If someone asks you to go unreasonably out of your way for them, when your oil is low, you will need to say 'no' or at least help them within the realm of certain limitations. *Not to put conditions on your giving or love for others,* but just try to balance how much energy you put out when your energy or *oil* is low.

Now back to being prepared. I encourage you to think ahead and do what you need to do to lower your stress, be prepared for set-backs and manage your limitations. You will need to make accomodations for your limitations. Know your triggers and manage them.

If your limitation is a chronic mental or physical disorder, then you will almost have to have your own set of rules and guidelines. Not to be a 'poor me, diva victim'... but once again, know yourself and manage your time, energy and activities accordingly.

Since most disease is triggered by some major stressor, then managing your daily stress is number one, even if you have to adopt strict habits. *If being late causes you stress, you may have to decide being an hour early for all engagements works for you.* And since the disease state is so complex, your personal rules may be different from others suffering from the same challenges... because your unique situation is just that, *unique.*

If your condition is chronic, and stress causes you to relapse, then having your own rules is key. It is imperative to know yourself... know your triggers and know what brings you peace. And, guess what? Know that those triggers may change as you change and grow. And what brings you peace one day, may not the next; *and vice versa.*

Sometimes when you have chronic fatigue and pain, and you find something or some place that brings you peace and you keep going back for more until you've smothered and sort of overused that outlet, you then discover that that outlet has now become your pain source. So, finding a healthy balance is what you're looking for! Be patient and kind to yourself and try a little balance.

If you have a loved one with a chronic mental or physical disorder, and you're so worried about them and determined to 'fix' them… sometimes your worry can do more harm than good. Try not to love with 'worry.' Since stress is the number one trigger for them, then your worry and stress is not going to help. So, find some peace and balance yourself. You need self-care too. The best you can do is be a peaceful example. Be a good listener, be flexible. Try not to give your opinion or advice unless you are specifically asked for it.

Now I know there are some severe cases out there and 'care-givers' seem to be the most overlooked. You need support and balance too… and reprieve from your roller-coaster ride as well.

So, when I speak of 'limitations', I am not just referring to one party.

Living A *Full-Life* With Our Limitations

For the rest of this section, when referring to *limitations*, I may also simply be referring to when we feel out of balance. So, no matter how big or small your imbalance, this section can refer to you as well. Living with any chronic limitation can leave us hopeless, so know that you can live a full-life, but at your own pace.

On Opposite Living

You may have to actually engage in "Opposite Living".

Work Smart, Not Hard

It seems, sometimes, that traditional society teaches: "work now, play later"… or "work hard, and it will pay off." Well, I believe everyday and every hour should be properly managed and lived at a healthy pace.

For me, when people come 'at me' with that 'work hard' motto, I freeze. The only way for me is to 'work smart'... not hard. Working with desperation, anxiety and mania only shuts down my mind and energy. So, whenever you feel overwhelmed, take a break, shift to another activity and come back to your work later. *Unless, of course, something is due and it is mandatory to finish it at that time.*

Do whatever you need to throughout the day to recharge and gain clarity, as long as it is safe and healthy. It also helps to be overly prepared for your endeavors, that way... those anxiety-filled co-workers or clients will not, as easily, overwhelm you.

Only you know what works for you. So, if 'working-hard' sends your body the wrong message, work smart. Calmness equals clarity and productivity.

Having clear intentions and goals with yourself and others helps with working 'smart' too. And learning to communicate those intentions effectively helps as well. If you realize you have taken on too much, know that it is ok to reestablish your goals. Cut back, communicate with others and do your best.

Be proud of yourself for not shutting down and falling back into another relapse. Learn to work smart!

Service Before Self or Self Before Service

Well, which is it? Tradition teaches, 'Service Before Self'… but in Opposite Living, I am going to address 'Self Before Service'.

Sure, we all know to put others first. But, you cannot give someone oil if yours is dangerously low. And, once again, I am not saying your giving should be conditional, but I am encouraging you to take care of yourself and know your limitations. As the airline stewardess says, "Put the oxygen mask on yourself first, please." You cannot help someone else if you are passed out on the floor.

I think society reminds us so much to put others first, that we forget the importance of balance and self-care. Give yourself permission for self-care… and sometimes, know that it is ok to say "no."

Once A Month or Once a Week

Even with limitations, we can still live a full service-oriented life like others, but with modifications. You may volunteer once a month instead of once a week. You may sign up as a 'back up' person for an event or committee. You may want to find an organization that will let you volunteer when only you are able to or available.

You may find that any weekly commitment is too much. Just in case you are in the middle of a relapse and need to back out on your weekly commitment, allow for these changes in your energy and schedule and find something that will give you flexibility, but not enable your weaknesses. I always find if I over commit myself and have to cancel, I feel worse about myself. So, under commit if that works for you.

You can participate in life… and creating your own version and level of participation still enables you to live a full life, but at your own pace, even if it's *once a month, and not once a week!*

Immediate Gratification, not Delayed

This next little section has to do with immediate instead of delayed gratification. It simply has to do with listening to your body. Tradition teaches us to practice discipline by living a life filled with delayed gratification. But, when you have a chronic condition, you better listen to your body and give it exactly what it needs when it needs it to prevent pain and a possible relapse.

When I am driving just an hour down the road, or sitting in church or in class, and I feel the slightest pain in my hips and back, I have to get up and stretch. If I try to remain still and think I should be disciplined or polite and stay seated; well, then it only gets worse. Since fibromyalgia is a soft tissue disorder, it is imperative to move when you feel ligaments and tissue tightening. Otherwise, the pain and tissue will get more stuck. The pain and overreaction of the tissue and symptoms are just like a really bad arthritis. But, luckily, it is not degenerative.

Once already in a relapse or flare-up… the body does not release itself from just one nights rest or one good stretch. It may take days or weeks for the body to reset itself back to normal. So, you must give your body exactly what it needs when it needs it.

Once you have recovered from your flare-up or relapse, then you may want to actually practice a little delayed gratification in certain areas of your life.

Small Goals

Living life with a disability, you may have to live life by a different set of rules and goals. You may have one set for the healthy you and another set for the 'fatigued' you. Set small goals, and be o.k. living them over and over again. Because, of course, the most important goal is prevention… to minimize your set-backs. Traditional environments may teach us to set large goals and keep moving forward. Well, in Opposite Living, your main goal is to live by small attainable goals and reward yourself for the tiniest of accomplishments. Since stress is the number one trigger for our challenges, then practicing small successes will eventually break the stress cycle and lower our chance for relapse. So try it, and good luck!

Boundaries… Guess what? Set them, and others will follow.

The Boundary Crosser

She will peer into your psyche and soul uninvited.
He will psychoanalyze you without an appointment.
They will process your thoughts before you even think them.

The Boundary Crosser

I used to think the only language pushy people understood was… '*pushy*.' And since pushy is all they understand, then I would push back. And, well, that only caused more friction, more stress.

So, I discovered, set a boundary or build a wall, and they will not be able to push past it. For example, if someone is pushing a large table across the room, and they hit a wall; well, they will have to stop. They cannot push any further.

But, if instead of hitting a wall, someone is on the other side of the table pushing back, they are only going to push harder.

So, when setting boundaries, be firm. Be direct. Do not give details. Do not share your very true excuses with them, they will only find ways to push around them.

You could simply not be available for someone who you are needing to set clearer boundaries with… or you could simply let them know you are just not able to give them your time right now. There are really nice, but firm ways to set boundaries.

Try it… save your energy, you deserve it. Setting firm, non-detailed boundaries; and living by them… could save you many exhausting days, weeks or years of your life.

Tithing With Limitations

Chronic problems can get us stuck in a severe self absorbed cycle, with no end in sight. When we are stuck in a perpetual victim mode, we really believe there is no way we could ever help someone else. There's no hope, no matter what.

But, God does want us to live a balanced and full life, no matter our limitations. The tiniest amount of time, money or talent, is tithing; as long as it is truly, from the heart giving. Just as God doesn't want us to *give* with some huge ROI expectation, he also doesn't want us to give out of worry or guilt. When we start to worry if we're doing enough or giving enough, then the giving then becomes about you and not the giving.

For years, I was so overwhelmed, sick and depressed, I gave nothing… not my time, money nor talent. I had no money to give and I was too exhausted and stressed to give anything else. I was stuck in a victim mode. However, when I regained hope, I realized I could offer my peaceful, loving prayers. And so I did!

There's always something to give, even if it's just a prayer. Also, often times on 'giving cards' there's a space titled "other amount", even if it's lower than the suggested amount, you can still give a tiny something. So, even if you're bankrupt and on unemployment, you may still be able to give $1.00... if not, give a prayer.

If you are completely broke and can give of your time, then give of your time. If you're unable to give your time because of chronic illness... you may be able to join a group that will let you participate when you are able or available. Do not be afraid to go at your own pace.

Now, if you are unable to give of your time or talent because of existing commitments, and you are healthy... and wealthy; well, then give financially. Even if you do not attend church regularly, you may be able to help out a significant amount financially.

In the Catholic faith, there is something called, "Almsgiving". It simply means doing something for someone without telling anyone about it. It's great! I am sure you probably do this naturally anyway. But I never knew it actually had a name, Almsgiving!

So, know your situation is unique. You can always give something; time, money, talent or prayers… and at your own pace. Do not give out of worry or guilt. Have fun and enjoy giving.

Try not to judge when you are giving. I have a friend who never gives to the homeless, pan handlers in the street. She says, "they will just go spend it on alcohol or drugs." Well, that's fine. She should give where she is comfortable giving. But remember, true giving holds no judgement. That homeless person can spend your monitary gift wherever he or she wishes. If he or she uses it to hurt himself further, that is on his conscience, between him and God. How do you know he didn't spend it in a positive way? You don't.

So, try not to judge yourself or others when giving. Enjoy giving… and remember giving is just that, giving!

Religion/Tradition & Limitations

I would like to make it clear that my suggestions on self-care and 'Opposite Living' are not meant to contradict any religious or traditional organizations' teachings! Some of us just need a little extra help with self-care and balance.

When I was a year or so into my RCIA program at the Catholic Church… I had more stressors, and many more set backs. And had a point during my journey that I was angry that my church didn't put more emphasis on self-care and managing chronic problems. I felt there was really no place for me in the Catholic Church or any traditional type organization or religion. I wanted to go back to only associating with places that could relate to my unique 'pace with grace' situation.

But, I then realized something that kept me on my journey. I realized that any major religion is going to need to express itself in a way that reaches the masses. And if they use a language that only reaches out to one population, then they would not be doing a very good job reaching everyone. If they only spoke my language or related only to my journey, then they would not be effectively sharing the word of Christ with the world. So, I stayed.

I now realize that each of us has a unique journey. For how would the branches of the tree of life, or the Body of Christ, be filled without our unique selves?

Healthy Tips & Reminders for Living With Our Limitations

Learn Healthy Communication... as to avoid unhealthy self-fulfilling prophesies.

Learning healthy communication is key to managing ourselves and relationships. It lowers and can almost eliminate stressful situations. But learning to communicate while managing chronic limitations is difficult. It is just too exhausting to communicate at times. We have to think things through and confront... and that is just too exhausting. It would be much easier if people could read our minds. But they cannot. And if they could, would you really want them to? Because they cannot, they may read you inaccurately.

So, for me, communication is key. It does help eliminate or lower stressful expectations from others and yourself. It saves you, in the long run, from trying to communicate once things are stressful. It is easier to put forth energy in the beginning, than putting out energy in the end to try and fix things.

My biggest suggestion is the following: Learn healthy communication as to avoid unhealthy self-fulfilling prophesies. I know when I am overwhelmed and exhausted, it is easy to slip into my 'poor me' mode. And 'poor me' is o.k. to an extent. But for me, it triggers more stress hearing my negative and intense expression of myself. I would much rather say I am not available if I know something is going to be too tiring. But then you have the problem of those folks who feel like you are being 'short' or abrupt. But if it causes you more stress to go into details, go ahead and be short and direct. Most people will appreciate it, rather than being excuse oriented or whiny.

Once sucked into the 'poor me' circle talk, sometimes, it triggers more pain, fatigue and frustration; therefore, setting up a negative spiral or self-fulfilling prophesy of your problems.

I am not talking about the occasional complaining or venting to friends and family… I am just trying to discourage you from making it your primary language.

Break the Pain Habit

When managing a chronic condition, I am sure you have noticed how many days, weeks or months you actually feel bad. And that you can count on one hand how many days in a month or year you actually feel good. Well, can you imagine what 'feeling bad' does to your body's cellular memory? Each cell in the human body has a memory… especially our muscles and joints and tissue. Our body is always trying to protect itself. Every single reaction, even if it is painful, at least has the good intention of protecting itself. I like to think of the human body like I do God. He wants us to survive and do our best and thrive… so he is constantly trying to make himself known and present to us. Well, the same is true for the human body. We are designed to survive and protect ourselves. So, this is a positive thing…but, most chronic illness is simply just a stress response that has gotten 'stuck'… or has just overworked itself. Think about addiction. We are just trying to escape our pain. Think about auto-immune disease. From my understanding, the body thinks there is an invader, so it attacks itself. We are trying so hard to protect ourselves and survive, that sometimes, the communication within our bodies gets miswired… like misunderstandings miscommunications. We are just human, so we are not going to do as good of a job protecting ourselves as God does making himself known to us.

So, back to the muscular and cellular memory… our bodies are so use to feeling bad, that it is, in essence, a stuck habit. It is not our fault and it is not like we can just break that habit. But, I will try to encourage you to find something that is safe, healthy and non-addictive that feels good. And you may have to retrain the body's memory by doing it over and over again. So, I am encouraging you to feed your mind and spirit as well as your body.

My escape from 'feeling bad' is my chiropractor, my church and prayer… and exercise. Do not be afraid to feel good. After I visit my chiropractor, I am in the floor for days… at least 5 times a day, stretching and breathing. I am trying to help my body let go of the 'out of alignment back' or the stuck shoulders or the stuck hip.

Make time to break the habit of pain… even if it is just for a little while. Do it long enough… and you may see some changes occur. Maybe you can try to feel good longer between your set backs. Some healthy activities I will refer to in this next section, *Healthy Distractions*.

Healthy Distractions

As I began to heal and move through my years of chronic fatigue syndrome and fibromyalgia… I learned that sometimes I simply need healthy distractions. For the first couple of years, I needed support. I needed to talk about my pain and problems and gain support that way. Talk about them until someone listened or acknowledged my pain. Well, after several years of that dynamic within myself and with others… I began to change. Talking about my pain and problems would trigger more pain. When I began to grow and change, others did not know to grow with me. So, I then learned, instead of focusing on the problem, it seemed to help to have healthy distractions. So, I tried to break the habit of talking about my problems, but it did not work. If a loved one or family member treated me or spoke to me in the same way they had been for years, I would have a sort of post-traumatic stress response to that nagging negative worry talk.

So, I stopped reaching out to others every time I felt like complaining…*I was trying to break the habit.* But, it only caused depression. And if I didn't have a healthy activity going on all the time, the down time would allow for me to fall back into the habit of feeling bad for feeling bad. It was almost like trying to break some sort of strange addiction. My body was use to the habit of feeling bad. So, I am encouraging you to, when you feel good, and have the energy, make a list of healthy activities. Because once you are already in a set back, you may not have enough mental energy to figure out what to do, you may not be able to think clearly enough to choose a healthy activity. So, make a list while you are healthy. Refer to that list when you are not healthy. Even have a little plan for each distraction. Because when you feel bad, you may not even remember how to execute that healthy activity. And these activities can be life savers, they distract us from the pain and frustration.

Some activities that work for me are the following:

Church, prayer group or bible study are spiritually and intellectually stimulating.

Meditation or breathing and stretching exercises, in case you are too physically tired to actually exercise.

Video games are a great brain and central nervous system distraction, once again, in case that is all you are able to do physically at that time.

Playing with your pet, fetch or catch.

Playing cards… even solitaire.

Pottery class, drawing class, writing class, photography class.

Even watching a performance or sporting event… going to the event to get out of the house and out of yourself.

Anytime you can help others, lots of nursing homes need visitors and volunteers.

Photo book and framing.

Reading a great novel.

Studying something new; history, Spanish, accounting.

Anyway, find the activities when you are feeling good and have a game plan to refer to when feeling bad.

Good luck and God Bless!

Pace With Grace

This is my favorite to live by. It is very simple… Pace… with Grace. Think this thought when you feel like overreacting to life. If you pause only for 20 seconds and repeat this phrase a few times and visualize God filling you with his grace at a nice steady pace, it really does help any situation!!

That's all. Pace… with grace.

Stay Away From 'Pain Pals'

I am not sure any other way to say this except, "stay away from pain pals." Have you ever found yourself in sort of a downward spiral verbal panic attack? And certain others around you, feed it? Maybe, at first, they want to help. Maybe they have the same problems. Maybe, initially, it is comforting to ramble and complain and have someone else relate to your pain.

It is actually nice to have support. But if your support has a worse addiction to pain than you, it may not be a great match. I am not saying dismiss them from your life. It is sometimes a blessing… like a mirror, but a reflection of your worst self. Kind of like a shadow.

So, if someone is sort of a reflection of some of your challenging traits, like staying focused too long on pain, then they are kind of a blessing, a reminder of your worst self. These reminders are necessary at times.

Now, you may even find pain pals who are just that... painful and toxic. They sort of subconsciously can only relate to others by comparing battle wounds. Well, stay away. You eventually begin comparing who is the biggest victim. Stay away from these types of pain pals. Try your best to use good judgement. We cannot always stay away from special people in our lives, but we can work to not get stuck in the pain pal connection.

So, please, past the point of a little bit of relating to others with pain… you do not need to get addicted to a pain pal.

Stay away from pain pals. Fear feeds… and you do not need to have very many pain pals.

Limitations Make Us Whole

It seems that even our limitations make us whole....

How would we know who we are and who we are not without them?

How would we know what to fix and manage without them?

How could we come full circle and help others in similar situations without them? In the long run, they help us. So, how can we, in turn help others?

So embrace this gift.... because whoever you are, completes that particular branch of the body of Christ.

No one else has the same journey to share with others.

God makes us whole with all these gifts, so embrace this gift, this gift of living with our limitations.

I believe courage is sort of that 'jumpstart' or
vessel
that fear needs to be converted into
something good.

When fear meets courage along its journey,
Once again, there's hope…

Hope for wholeness, hope…
for true conversion.

For courage is the vessel
through which fear moves and comes out
on the other side, well-healed.

On Wholeness and Holiness…

"No child is perfectly whole in mind, body, spirit ability, nor can any child meet all of a parents' hopes and expectations, yet there is a wholeness of each and every child, a wholeness that is unique and brings with it a unique set of possibilities and limitations, a unique set of opportunities for fulfillment."

Fred Rogers (Mr. Rogers)

"Life can be lived to the fullest; no matter our limitations... we just need others to take us by the hand and walk with us. This is what they do at Sanctuary House... this is what you have done for me... and so I thank you once again and want you to know that we all have our own unique wholeness and holiness to reach... so, never ever stop reaching... God is there, you don't have to reach very far. The fog will lift... and this too shall pass." Georgianna Penn

"It's a choice we make
To make everyday a new beginning,
To make everyday a progressive step
towards our best selves."

The 12th Gift

"The Gift of Conversion"

There's always a chance for change,
A new beginning… conversion.
It isn't always an event,
or a date on a calendar.

It's not always
Some concrete goal we've achieved,
Nor is it graduation,
a new job or a move
across the country.

And neither is it an escape from ourselves
Or an addiction to the new.
It's a step we take within ourselves
And with God.

It's a choice we make
To make everyday a new beginning,
To make everyday a progressive step
towards our best selves.

A new beginning or conversion…

is not something
we wait to do "when"
It's a daily conscious effort
To stop living in the unconscious
Realm of ourselves…

To stop living in the past…
And worrying about the future.
To stop living in our pain, but rather
Move through it… to the other side.

It's a Gift God gives us
to live fully in the present moment.
God isn't sitting up there in Heaven with a
Checklist of our rights and wrongs.
He is a loving God… He is a forgiving
God.

And that is why he gave
his only Son, Jesus Christ.
To save us from ourselves…
For the Gift of Life and Love…
For the Gift of Conversion.

G. Penn Jan. 28, 2006

Healing Essays of the Heart

Above all else, guard your heart... for it is the wellspring of life."

Proverbs 4:23

Heart – "The heart is the dwelling place where I am … The heart is our hidden center, beyond the grasp of reason and of others; only the Spirit of God can fathom the heart and know it fully. The heart is the place of decision , deeper than our psychic drives. It is the place of truth, where we choose life or death. It is the place of encounter, because as image of God we live in relation: it is the place of covenant." *Catholic Catechism. See Source Notes.*

Reconciliation to Resurrection

A Recovery of Heart

From darkness to light, from bondage to freedom, purgatory to paradise, reconciliation to resurrection… we've all been there in some way or another. Unmanaged stress, unhealed wounds and anger, resentment, guilt and fear can all manifest negatively into our core being; not only physically, but spiritually as well. Once the spirit has been shaded, there is very little fuel left for the rest of ourselves.

Stress and sin can paralyze us spiritually, mentally, and emotionally, and if left unprocessed can manifest into physical pain or illness. Physiologically, our body's sole purpose is to survive, and stress can leave our bodies running and screaming for help; therefore, creating more stress. Confused and helpless, the body/mind creates coping mechanisms for protection from that original stressor. Coping mechanisms that can then become negative patterns of chronic fatigue and pain, chronic worry and depression, addiction or illness… and therefore, piling on more layers of stress keeping us further from our God and true selves.

So, if the body's sole purpose is to survive… and house the Spirit; and the Spirit's soul purpose is to love and provide life, and God is love and love is life. Then isn't it through this renewal of the spirit, this reconciliation of the heart, this intimate connection with our God that leads to a much healthier and peaceful survival?

The sooner we name our stressor or stressors, the sooner we can work with God to mend our impurities and make room for true life and love. We get out of our own way and out of God's way… and only then can we experience true healing.

Once we experience this transformation, we can then be made an empty shell for God's grace to shine through out onto others and out into the world.

To lay down our burdens to God, to seek peace and reconciliation with all our hearts brings not only a renewal of the Spirit, but a renewal of the entire body, mind, spirit and soul…

When we take one step towards God… God takes many, many millions of steps towards us.

Written April 24th, 2005 Inspired by the Holy Spirit, St. Pius X Catholic Church & staff, the beautiful music of St. Pius, by my family & friends, by all of life's experiences good and bad. Thank you St. Pius for showing me the true Holy Grail.

"Anthropology of the Spirit"

As human beings, our main purpose or goal is to survive and procreate. One must survive in order to procreate, and one must procreate in order to survive.

As spiritual beings, this same goal holds true. We must survive so that we can procreate God's love here on Earth… we must procreate love in order to survive in God's eternal kingdom.

To reach this ultimate goal of salvation, it starts with each of us everyday. To share God's love, to live in peace and harmony with one another, not only prepares us for eternity, but also makes our stay here on Earth a much more pleasant experience.

If our goal here on Earth is to share God's light and love, and be the best we can be so that we may help others be the best they can be, then don't we owe it to our God and to ourselves to survive the best we know how?

We owe it to our God to know who we are, know our strengths, know our weaknesses, manage our stress, use our unique gifts and talents in accordance with God's will…

encourage others, bring love, be love… and share love.

And since we are here on Earth as 'human' beings, and God has given us the responsibility to house the spirit within our human selves; then, we must equally respect and care for our human-selves as well as our spirit selves. And we must not only esteem ourselves, but equally esteem others as well. God is love… and "God wants us to balance our love for self and others,"… not to be self-centered, not to be others centered… but to be God-centered.

Treating ourselves and others with love and respect while nurturing all aspects of the human and spirit condition is the key to survival… both here on Earth… and in Heaven.

Written by Georgianna Penn… May, June, July of 2005 Inspired by the Holy Spirit, St. Pius the Tenth, my loving pastor, my loving sister, V.V., my friend, Alicia, all my loving family and friends and the healing power that surrounds 2210 North Elm St. Special thanks to the St. Joseph's Prayer Group.

"Purgatory and Paradise"

The garden was filled with many flowers and I was one of them. Some were petunias and others were pansies. Some were roses and some were wild flowers. I was a Wild Flower. I was growing prosperously and maturing along with the other flowers. I liked it here in the garden and I enjoyed my life. I was happy here.

However, I took this carefree life in the garden for granted. One evening, late in the month of August, I was picked. My master cut me and picked me right out of the garden. I was flattered. He loved me and cherished me with all his heart. He kept me in a beautiful bright green vase in the kitchen window sill. He watered me… and gave me sunlight. He gave me everything I wanted except the freedom to venture back to the garden to see my friends. He told me, "your friends will always be there. You don't need to go back to visit."

He always wanted me nearby. There close to him, I made him happy. He told me I was the best flower he had ever picked. I knew he truly loved me and never wanted to be without me. This passion was flattering too. No one ever wanted to spend so much time with me before, not even in the garden.

After a few months, in the bright green vase, I felt strange, I felt alone. "What's the matter?" He would ask. "Oh nothing," *I would plead.* I felt suffocated. What was I to do? I was slowly dying. But why? I missed the joyful garden; I missed the freedom of interacting with the other flowers. How could I be so discontented with someone who loved me so dearly?

I often explained these horrible feelings to him. He offered only more suffering and conflict. The more I wanted freedom, the tighter he squeezed. The more I wanted sunlight, the more he shaded me. However, the more water I wanted, the more he gave me, almost to the point of drowning. Pure honesty did no good; he did not respect my feelings. I felt lifeless; I was drained; he had cut off my support system.

"I give you everything, Wild Flower, so why your misery? I give you water, I give you love. No one will ever love you as I do."

Trapped in that bright green vase, I looked out at the world afraid I would never be a part of it again. I had stopped growing. My poor green leaves were wilted and shabby.

I knew I was dying from the inside out. It was painful. My master said to me, "You are sick Wild Flower; why are you sick?"

"If you truly loved me, you would have left me in the garden to grow instead of picking me to keep all for yourself. You have stopped my life and now I am going to die. If only you had allowed me to remain in the garden instead of taking me into your lair to be smothered."

I was dead. I awoke in a new garden; one I had never experienced before. The sky was a beautiful hue of blue. The sunlight was of great radiance. The smell of wild flowers all around me inspired my blossoms to new growth.

Was I dead… or was it just that mere piece of my past that had passed away? Whatever it was, I knew I was alive again.

Whatever is holding us hostage… whether it's a job, a relationship… or merely a thought process… always have hope and know that at anytime, our blossoms can be inspired to new growth. Through patience, love and faith we are renewed. Through Christ, we can live again.

Written at Greensboro College in 1992. Published in the "Lyre" – Greensboro College Creative Arts Magazine… April 15th 1992.

The Many Other...
Peaces & Places of God

Thank you Madison Presbyterian Church for your spiritual and moral foundation!

Thank you to my childhood minister and all the congregation for many great years at MPC!

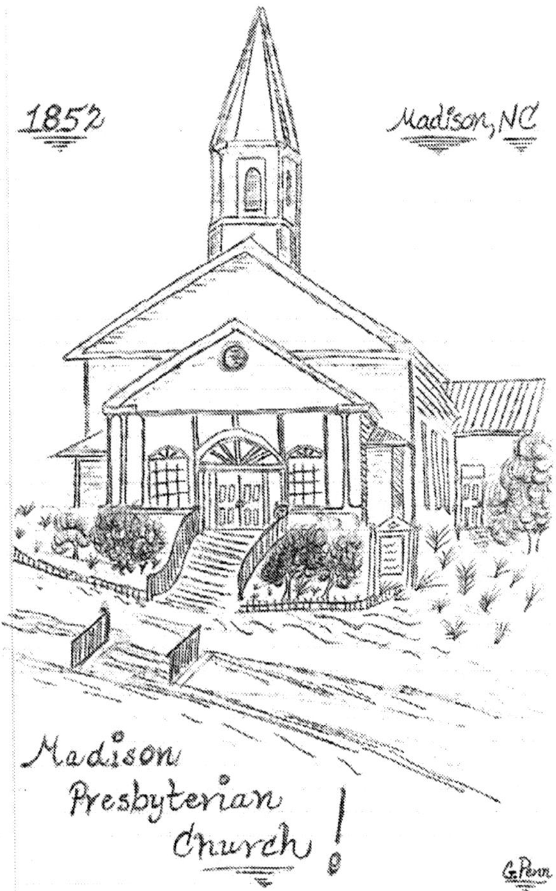
1852
Madison, NC
Madison
Presbyterian
Church!
G. Penn

Thank you St. Pius for your spiritual CPR... and for being that light to which I am drawn over and over and over again!

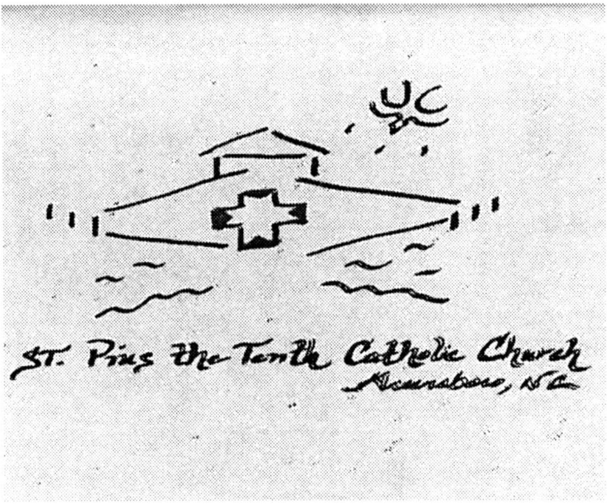
St. Pius the Tenth Catholic Church

Thank you Unity for your perpetual self-help program. You are so loving and accepting of everyone. We love you Unity!

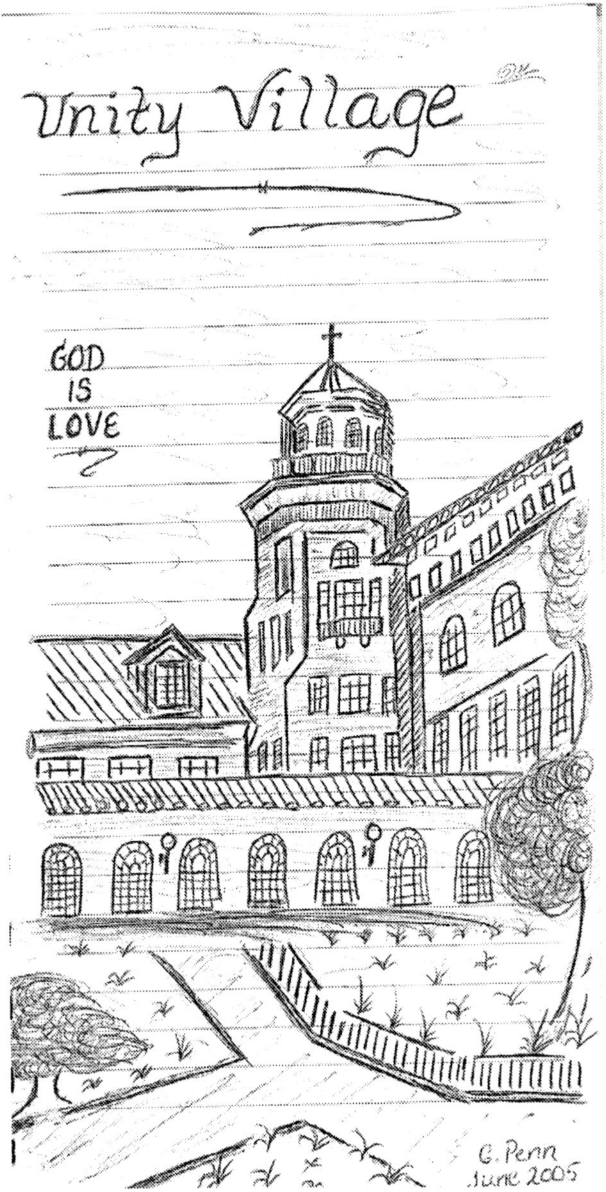
Unity Village
GOD IS LOVE
G. Penn
June 2005

Thank you Eucharist. There are no words great enough... just being in your presence is almost too much! Thank you Eucharist!

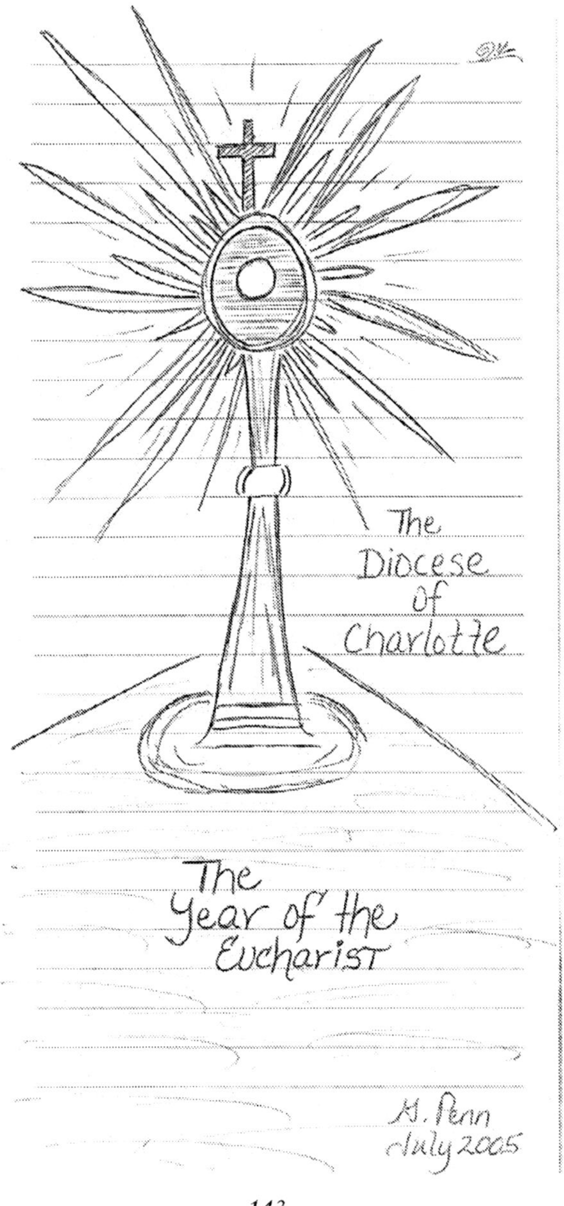
The
Diocese
of
Charlotte
The
Year of the
Eucharist
G. Penn
July 2005

Thank you Duke for being that perfect escape from the day! And thank you for watching over Grandma 'A'.

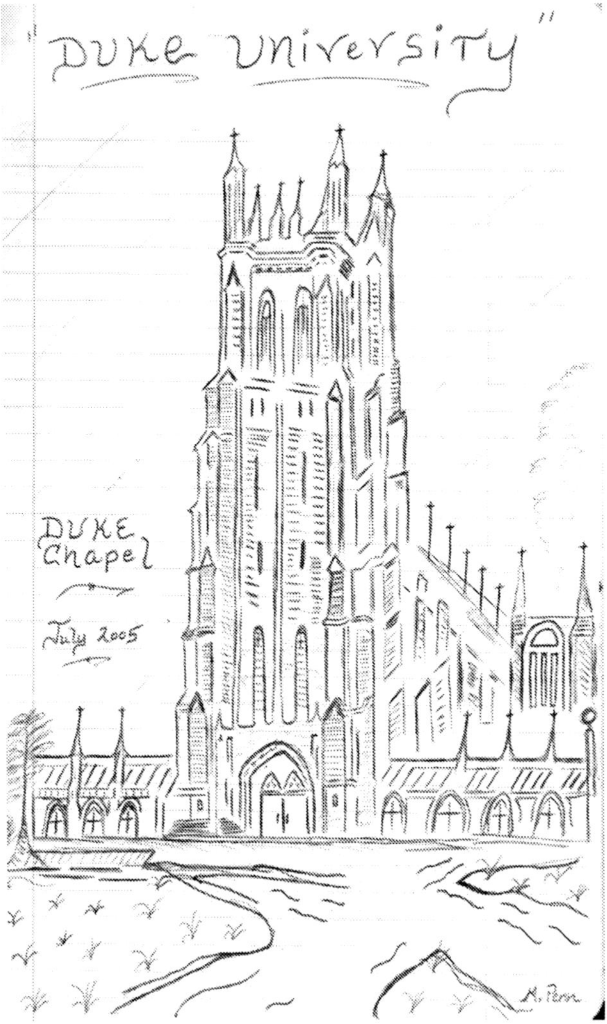
"DUKE University"
DUKE Chapel
July 2005
M. Penn

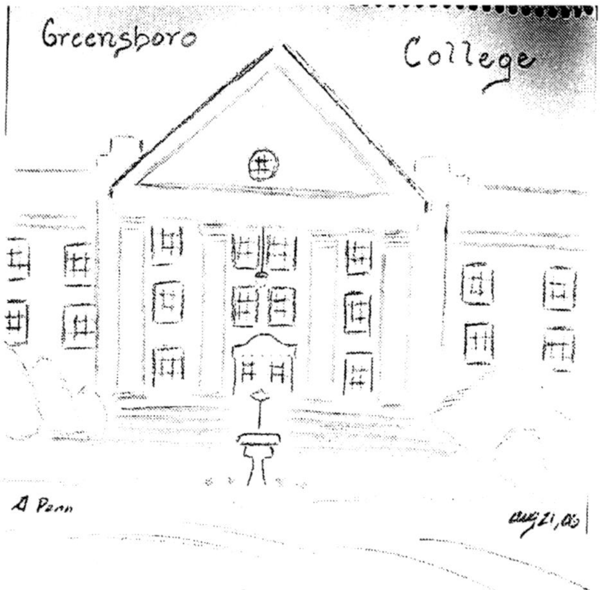

- 1838 -

Thank you Greensboro College for teaching me the beautiful art of creative writing... thank you for providing me with a place where I could truly self-actualize.

You were the best years of my life... so far!

Thank you home. Once again, there are not enough words. You are my foundation... I still love coming home to the most beautiful B&B *in the world!*

I love you mom and dad. I love you Madison.

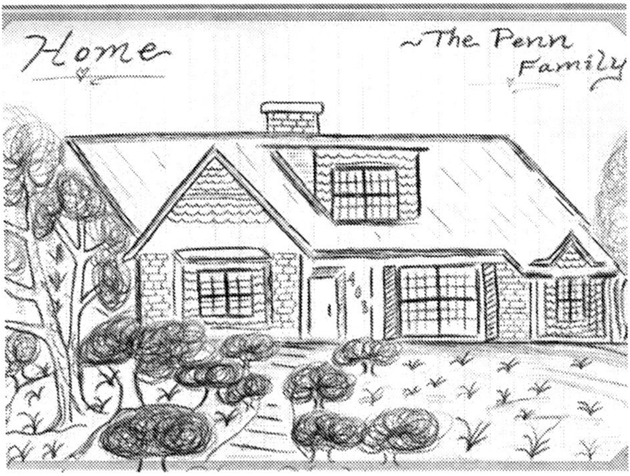
Home
~The Penn Family

Thank you St. Francis for building your prayer center in my hometown!

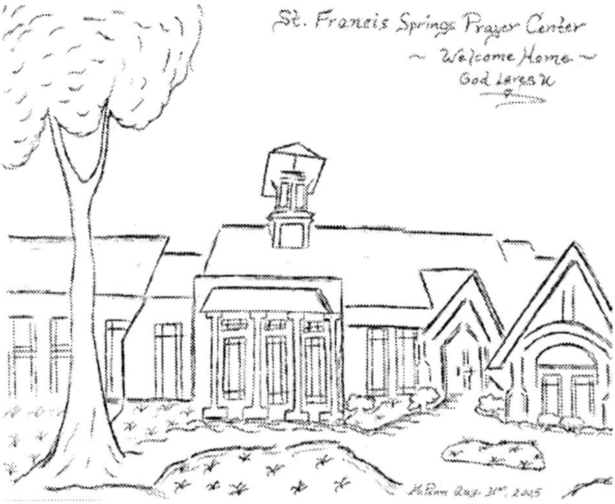
St. Francis Springs Prayer Center
~ Welcome Home ~
God Loves U

Thank you Kerry and Brad for the most beautiful day of my life... and yours too, I'm sure!

Thank you St. Gabriel for the art of communication and self-expression.

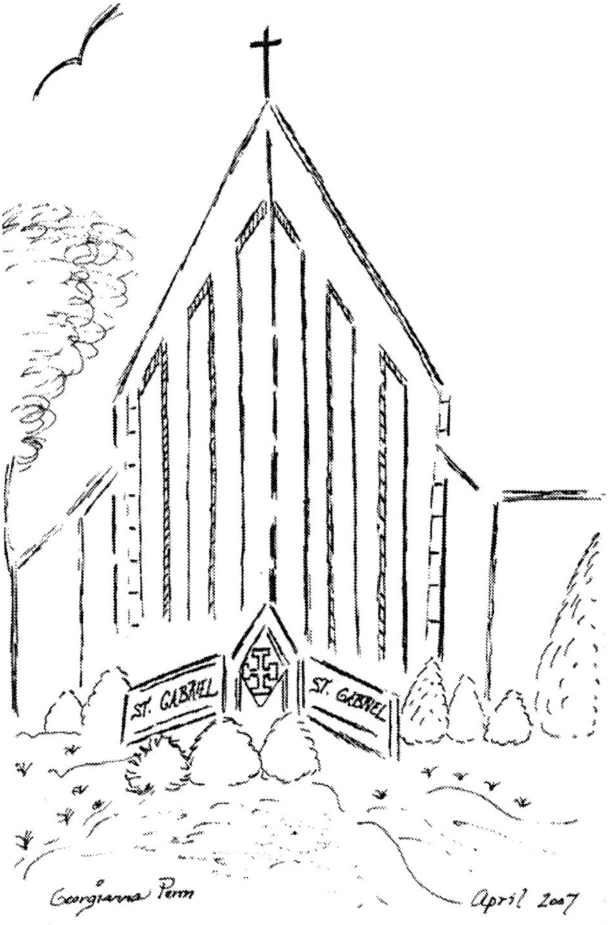
ST. GABRIEL
ST. GABRIEL
Georgianna Penn
April 2007

Thank you Vaughanie for our wonderful memories. We are so lucky to have each other and it is 'Almost Perfect' here!

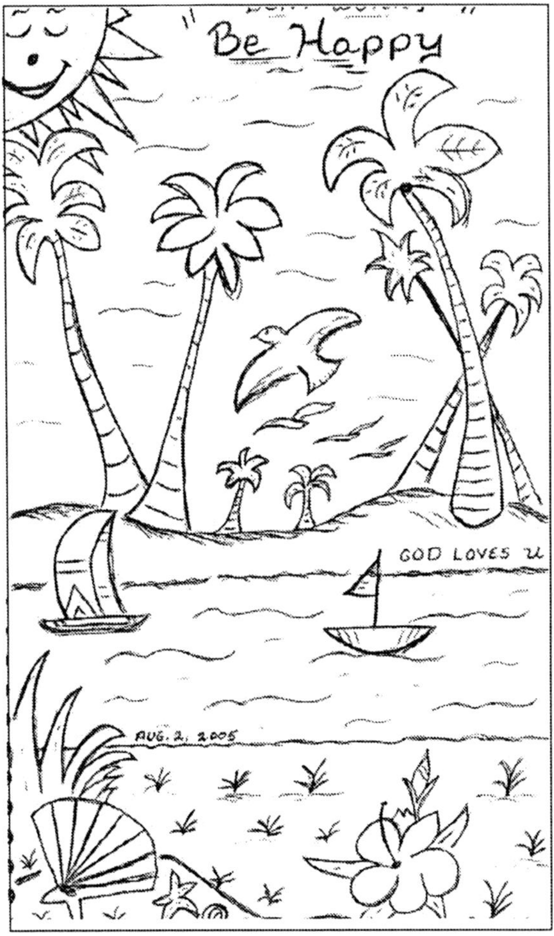
"Be Happy
GOD LOVES U
AUG. 2, 2005

Full Circle of Grace

I now take you on a journey through the 12 Gifts of Grace towards your own unique wholeness with the Full Circle of Grace workbook.

Prayer – The Soul's Intervention - Through words, actions, rituals, silence, song and dance… we all have different ways of prayer.

Option One: This section allows you to journal for one week, keeping up with the different ways you pray. You could make notes on the different types of prayer for your many different moods and needs and needs of others. Write letters of thanksgiving to God… or letters of blessings and thanksgiving to others. Keep in your journal, or share with others or share at a prayer group.
Option Two: If you are working with a prayer group or with someone… practice your prayers of thanksgiving, of song, of prose… or of giving and receiving. Organize an hour of community prayer in a structured layout... Here is an example: Feel free to create your own structure.

Opening prayer – *Our Father or Hail Mary* or something everyone knows and can say together.
Prayers of Thanksgiving – Each of you name two things you are thankful for in this moment. This week, month or year, whatever structure you choose.
Prayer of song or prose – Each of you choose a song or poem… or both. If it is music, teach one another and sing together.
Scripture or Spiritual Reading – Choose a bible verse or teaching… or any other spiritually

inspired reading… and reflect.

Intercessory Prayers – Prayers of need… for others, for yourself… or any other need… keep these prayers silently in your hearts or speak them out loud. Keep them short or detailed… whatever you feel drawn to do.

Prayer of song or prose – End group with song or poem or reading.

Leader of prayer group or each member ends with one more thank you and blessing for the week to come.

Have fun, be blessed and good luck!

Guardian Angel Prayer

Hail Mary
Our Father
Nicene Creed
Unity Prayer
Song
Song

Art – The Soul's Expression – Through art, music, dance, our love of a hobby... teaching, creating and sharing in any expressive and healthy activity... is food for the soul!! In this section, keep a journal and list everything that brings you joy, peace and freedom from the day's stress. Anything that gets you lost in the flow of the spirit and fills your soul.

I believe the soul's expression is not competitive... art, music, poetry... any healthy expression from your soul is simply that ... The Soul's Expression!!

Have fun and many blessings. Make a pact with a friend to practice these expressions weekly or daily with others, with yourself, or in a class... whatever works for you. Or just share with someone weekly what you've created or accomplished. You may have accomplished an activity, or goal, a piece of art, a song or poem... or you may have simply found a special place to sit-down, stretch, relax and let go.

Try some of these or create your own!

Sketch words of inspiration in big bubble letters.
Make a homemade greeting card for someone.
Buy some molding clay and create a new soothing shape each day.
Write down inspirational quotes you read or hear.

Write down your own inspirational quotes.
Write a song or poem… even if it is silly. Get it out, express it!!
Find a yoga class or any other exercise that appeals to you.
Find a park or special place to sit and meditate or walk.
Play with your pet or child or play a board game with your neighbor or roommate or spouse.
Play an instrument.
Write down everything you are grateful for from that week.

Whatever you do, give yourself permission to let go and feel peace and love.

If you are overwhelmed and cannot figure out what to do… or have forgotten how to relax, how to have fun or feel good… try something new and different. Go into a store or church you have never been into before, even take yourself bowling, or to a movie… or just drive to another city. Even driving down a road in your own town you have never been down before, can shift you out of yourself. Look what it did for me!! Just changing your physical location for a moment can shift you into being open to inspiration. Just be safe and make sure it is healthy and safe for you and others. Have fun and God bless!

Hope – The Soul's CPR - The tiniest flicker of hope can give us the strength to make it through. Who in your life, has inspired you and given you hope? Who have you given hope to?

Make a list each week of the situations or people who have given you hope for the day or moment. Make a list of those signs and synchronicities that give you hope throughout the day. Put this in your journal along with the other responses to these 12 steps… share or keep to yourself.

Think of those situations that still cause you stress and think of how you can regain hope and write down your own hope to yourself.

Have fun and God Bless!

Love Your Shadow – Love and Honor all parts of yourself. You are who you are. So, turn those seemingly limitations into strengths and gifts… find the positive in every aspect of yourself. If you are obsessed with numbers and bills and keep adding up your debt or bills each week and not really moving forward… find another way to use this strength of "adding up numbers". Instead of beating yourself up for this obsession… or trying to stop the behavior… volunteer to help someone else with their bills and budget and see how yours easily falls into place. Take that same trait and volunteer or get a part time job using that gift. Or just re-direct it to another type task.

However, doing an opposing behavior sometimes does help… just find what works for you. Find a healthy and safe outlet for all parts of you. Sometimes, when I get stuck in emotion, it helps to do something linear or opposite of the emotion… add up numbers, learn a song, go to a group class setting and focus on a task together… and snap out of the stuck emotion.

There are beautiful gifts to be found in all parts of yourself, so don't ever put yourself down or feel bad for a specific trait… I bet there is a healthy outlet just around the corner.

If you are a procrastinator… instead of staying stuck and trying so hard to start a project and can't, do anything. Society sometimes teaches delayed gratification… or do the difficult homework first… Well, for me, it took many years of turmoil to realize that sometimes… doing the easiest thing first, gets my energy, brain and confidence flowing… It's like a warm-up for the more difficult activity. So, I give you permission to do the most comfortable and easiest homework first… or, whatever works for you.

Make a list of your traits… good and bad… try not to use judgement words… just list them… Then either come up with a solution to improve or make that trait a comfortable trait or find another outlet for that trait.

Find the positive and don't take yourself too literally.

It's Only Love that Heals – Have you ever found yourself obsessed with work, exercise, church, therapy... almost like an escape... thinking, "well, with enough exercise... or if I just work, work, work, or go to more therapy or ... then I can fix me. Or I will be happy... when. Well, no matter how much you throw yourself into work, exercise, therapy... or whatever, without love, you may still find yourself out of balance. If you do not have a significant other or spouse... there's always the tiniest expressions of love and kindness in our daily lives.

Try the following: Be kind to your neighbor, send your parents or an elderly relative flowers or a nice greeting card. Try a little more kindness and encouragement at work. With a client or co-worker, give them a compliment or some encouragement. Just remember, no matter how hard you try to be happy or fix yourself... with love, all is better. Be patient and kind to yourself and others.

Each Other - Who has inspired you? Teachers, pastors, siblings, parents, friends? Write them a letter of gratitude! Good luck and have fun.

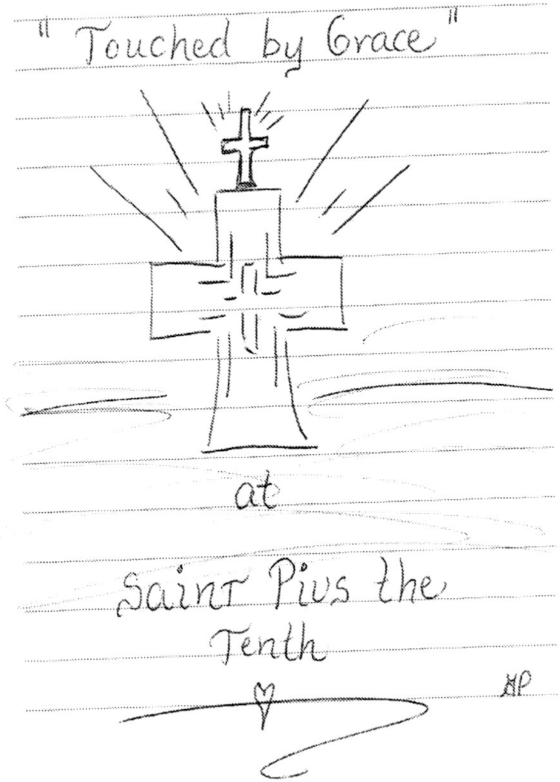
"Touched by Grace"
at
Saint Pius the
Tenth
MP

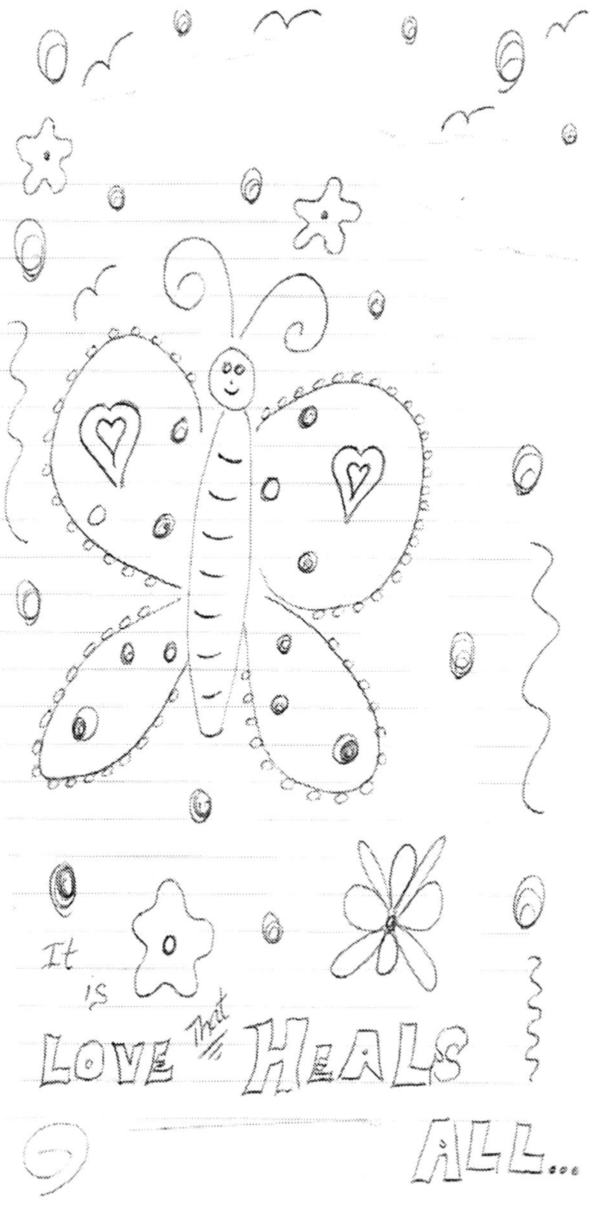
It
is
LOVE that HEALS
ALL...

Compassion – Sometimes compassion is not about understanding someone else's trials… but about showing them love and support whether we understand their situation or not. Who has shown you compassion? Who can you call today and share some compassion with… even if you don't fully understand their situation. An even greater challenge would be to call a friend or relative whose situation is actually puzzling or bothersome to you… and just listen and show some compassion without any judgement. Take yourself out of the picture just for a moment. Try it and keep it in your journal or share at a prayer group when discussing compassion. You and your prayer group could even focus on compassion for just one month… and cite times when your mentors or favorite leaders have shown compassion. Maybe use the New Testament in the Bible and find times when Jesus showed compassion. You can have compassion for those to whom you can relate and to those to whom you cannot. Good luck and have fun.

Love - Write out a definition or mission statement of what love means to you. Each week, write down two action steps you can take to help live out this mission statement.

Write them down and live them out.

Make sure it covers your loved ones as well as strangers or co-workers or neighbors… the activities should be different for these categories. Loving, but appropriate boundaries for each category. The co-workers or neighbors may be a simple act of kindness… or simply making a pact with yourself to communicate in a more respectful way with a co-worker or roommate or sibling, even if they are overreacting or stressing out on you. You can manage your reactions to stressful situations without letting someone walk all over you.

Write down your mission statement first and the actions will naturally follow!!!

You may refer to the book of Corinthians!

Faith – Family or group activity. In a group of 4 or more… each person has a partner. Place items on the floor… small trash cans, boxes, magazines, coke bottles, etc… sort of make an obstacle course. Cover your partners eyes with a handkerchief or bandana. Tie your partners hands loosely. You are then to guide your partner through the obstacle course by giving them verbal commands. Do not let them touch any of the items with their body… especially their feet. This is fun and a great trust building activity for teams, co-workers, roommates, friends, families or spouses.

Gratitude –

Keep a glass jar or small box by your front door or at your kitchen table or desk. You can paint the outside of it with uplifting words or quotes. Keep a small note pad by the jar or box. Everyday write down two things for which you are grateful.

Every few days, or at the end of the week, read aloud with a friend. Read at prayer group or with a friend, roommate, spouse or child or co-worker! Awesome! And have fun!

Courage

Courage is the active component of hope, love and faith. Courage, sometimes, is just 'fear' converted.

When, have you finally taken the steps needed towards a certain goal or change?

Write a letter to yourself congratulating yourself for the steps you took… and write down a continued plan of courage for that particular issue, or similar issues… or just life in general.

Good luck and have fun.

Invite a friend to be your 'courage sponsor.' Ask them to observe and listen. Ask them to coach you only if you want their 'tough love' and coaching… if not, just having them observe or witness your journey, is plenty!

The Gift of Conversion – Make a list of moments of conversion for you… in a relationship, in your life… or just throughout your day or week. Maybe just a thought process shifted to a more freeing and positive one. Maybe you have worked really hard on a change… leaving an unhealthy situation, and maybe each baby step was a form of conversion for you. Or maybe it is as clear as graduation, confirmation or your wedding day. In the Christian faith, it is believed that if we live our lives based on the teachings and truths of Christ, we can continuously be converted daily here on Earth and after death. So, with this in mind, we need not continue to live in the past nor stay stuck in worry or regret and fear. It is actually an insult to our higher self and our God. So, if you find yourself stuck in this negative addiction of regret, worry and fear… find a friend or something to distract you from yourself. Again, it could be a person, place, ritual/healthy daily activity that brings you back into the present and converts you right back to your healthy self. So, keep a journal and adopt a daily ritual or activity. My conversion activity for this month is to make a scrap book and picture frame of my best friends wedding. Each day and moment I work on it, I feel a peace of my healthy, happy self return to me. And my daily ritual is to say daily affirmations as I awake each morning until I feel a clear mental shift. My weekly ritual is to go to a different mass at my church as to meet new people… and go into a different cute retail store each week, one I have never been to before. Sometimes a weekly ritual may be to go to my hometown or to my hometown church as to reconnect with that part of myself. You can find whatever works for you… and switch it up each week!

Good luck and have fun.

More poems

of peace and inspiration

Peace and Inspiration

Praise yourself
and others often.

Seek to be with those
who build you up, support
you and love you.

Never let anyone's skepticism,
concerns or negativity
diminish your spirit and soul.

Let the art of life flow,
and live it with
grace, dignity and joy.

Written in Williamsburg, Va.
With sister, Liz!

Peace and Balance

Find balance
and fill your cup
daily with that which
soothes your soul.

Say "I love you" often
And seek to find
Peace
In all situations.

Keep your dreams alive
And never stop
finding
The beauty
In everyday life.

Poems written summer 2006

What Does God Look Like?

When I was a little girl, I had a vision of what God looked like. My vision consisted of my Presbyterian minister, Harold; our neighbor, Mr. Rodenbough and our friend, Mr. Wall. I came to discover that I was right. These three wise men are so loving and kind, that *yes*, this is what God looks like. To this day, they are still dear friends of ours… and I love them. Their peaceful essence and solid white hair tends to help portray the very essence of God.

My vision today of God is simple. When I look straight above to the blue skies and white puffy clouds, I think of God. I picture him up there with a big smoke machine, like the ones used in Hollywood. And he is blowing out beautiful and creative shapes. And no two shapes are alike, but all are beautiful and unique in their own way… and they all compliment and sort of support one another. And I think this is how he creates us and wants us to live… in unity with one another, complimenting and supporting one another with our own unique, God-given strengths and beauty.

What Does God Smell Like?

Well, besides the green grass in my parents huge back yard, I think of the beauty, purity and happiness of God when I smell the incense and oils used in my Catholic church. They are so intoxicating.. I am not sure why they are used on some days rather than other days at mass, but they smell so pure and peaceful, like God!

In the Catholic faith, many things are used as to allow us to experience God through all of our senses. The stained glass and statues, allow us to experience him visually. The incents and oils allow us to smell his purity. The music, the readings and the prayers allow us to hear the word of God… and the Eucharist allows us to taste and live the word and very essence of God.

Everyone, whether you are Catholic or not, should experience a Christmas Eve or Easter Vigil service at St. Pius sometime in their lifetime… it's just magical!

What does God look like to you? What smells bring you peace. What sights fill you with awe? Maybe it is just the sight of seeing someone being kind to another… or maybe it's the sound of your family and friends getting together celebrating. Think about keeping a list of how God touches your life everyday in every possible way. And write it down and share your thoughts with loved ones or at a prayer group. Have fun and God Bless!

St. Puis X
Catholic Church

"Making a Place at the Table"

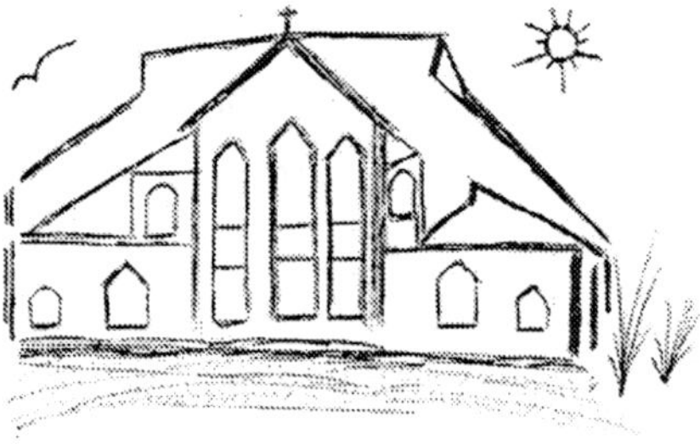

We Can't Grow

Without Help From You

I love this church, indeed I do.
For it was made for me and you.
I love this church, yes I do.
But it is growing… and multiplying too.
I love this church, indeed I do, but it can't grow
without help from you.
I love this church, this I know.
But we need a place where your daughter can go.
I love this church, this is true, but we need a place
for her daughter too.
I love this church, yes I do. But we need your
pledge,
so we can start our building anew.
I love this church, but it is true…
That we can't grow
Without help
From you.

Please call your builder today… or place your pledge card in the collection basket at mass, or drop it off at our Parish office. Just a note from your St. Pius Capital Campaign builders!

June 2007 G. Penn

I Saw a Rainbow and Thought of Jack

Driving home today, I saw a rainbow…
And thought of you.

I had just received news that you were ill and
feeling blue.
However, I had a meeting at McMichael High,
And had briefly forgotten that my friend,
Jack, was about to fly.

But driving down 220, crossing Horse Pen
Creek…I saw a rainbow and began to think.

The colors were perfect… red, green, and blue.
And time stood still, with beautiful thoughts
Of you.

I turned around, in the middle of Battleground and
began to drive north… and thought,

"not a great time for a visit, but there's no turning
back…"
Because I saw a rainbow… and thought of my
friend, Jack.
With no gift in hand, no flowers, no card… all I
had to give,
Was a little peace of me… and my pocket Rosary.

See, I'm not Catholic, and neither are they, but
Jack was there… when I first learned… to pray.

He sang in the choir, I admired him so. He made
me feel safe… and loved, I know.

I always felt happy when I thought of Jack… for
he even taught me to swim, while towing me on his
back.
He's shared his love, his talents, his smiles… and
taught us all to scrub his blue pool tiles.

"Sweet little Jesus Boy" would be proud… for he
has you, on his team now.

You've filled us with your song, your style, your
charm.
You've filled us with laughter, kindness… and no
harm.

We will miss your smile, your song, your charm.
This, I'm sure.

So… when you see a Rainbow,

Think of Jack…
For it may be his soul…

Smiling, right back.

Written May 9 & 10, 2007

Written for my friend, Jack Sealy, who loved and lived life to the fullest… with all his heart… all his mind… and his whole soul.

Thank you Jack for being a part of my life, we will miss you.

Letters of Grace

Closing Prayer

I just realized my journey is not necessarily about becoming Catholic. If I become Catholic along the way… then, wow, that would be great, *like an extra, unexpected blessing!* In the beginning of this book, I stated that this book is not necessarily about religion or Christianity. But, I've now realized this book is all about Christianity; *peace, acceptance, love and hope.*

This book is my prayer to you.

Acceptance. My prayer for you is acceptance. Accept others where they are on their journey. Do not force or push your views or ways on others, especially your fears.

If someone finds peace meditating by a stream, but does not attend church regularly, they are no less closer to God because they are not part of a church community. I am no closer to God now that I have found a church. However, it does bring fullness and ritual to what I believe, kind of like finding that perfect soul mate with whom to spend the rest of your life. Or, like… you will always be close to your family and friends, but when you get together in celebration, it brings a little more wholeness and fullness to your relationship. So, accept others where they are on their journey, whether they pray by a stream or by an altar.

My prayer for you is *peace.* Bring peace and respect to all of your interactions. Parents, do not fight in front of your kids. It splits the psyche and soul for everyone involved. Children respect your parents, especially as they age… *they're only getting smarter and wiser anyway!* Take responsibility for your relationships. Talk to each other, not about each other. And listen. *Listening* is the most precious and peaceful gift you can give someone.

Grace, my prayer for you is grace… *social grace.* Manage your stress, your actions and your reactions. *Past the point of occasional 'venting',* do not put your fears, anxiety and delusions on others.

Love, my prayer for you is love. Living a life and heart filled with love can automatically cause us to live by God's laws, without even consciously knowing what they are. The Ten Commandments have a way of putting themselves on autopilot when fueled by a heart filled with love.

Hope. My prayer for you is hope… that you will share hope with others. Someone once shared the tiniest bit of hope with me when I so desperately needed it. And, sometimes, that is all it takes to guide us away from an unhealthy path. *The tiniest flicker of hope* can be just enough to spark someone down a brighter path…a path that leads to hope, love and light… a path that leads to *faith.*

Once again, accept others. Do not condemn someone because they do not speak the language of Christ. For, they may be living the very essence and principles of Christianity, and not even know it!

Many Blessings to You!

Thank you to my 'Loving Sponsors'

Thank you to my 'Loving Sponsors' who paid for the publishing and initial printing of this book! Thank you so much for your donation… you were my "jumpstart"…

Thank you ***Helen Houston*** for always being right there as a loving support for me and my family's ventures… you were my first book sponsor! Thank you for being so nice to me at mass! All that time, I did not know your name, I certainly didn't know I already knew you?!! You are precious!

Thank you ***Cindy and Lloyd Hartsell***… Cindy, you are such a shining light… you are a true angel. Thank you for all the "hand-me-downs" over the years! Lloyd and your mom… and all of Charlotte are so lucky to have you close by at all times. Lloyd, you are the funniest, most charming, adorable and "hottest" dude in Charlotte! I am so glad you and Cindy have tied the knot!!! I hope you build and sell lots of new homes in Myers Park… your work is so beautiful!

Thank you ***Margot*** for being a loving sponsor for my book and always making me smile and feel so good about myself! You have a beautiful family, thank you for being in our lives!

Thank you ***Curt Bennett***… you are so kind and good. I have such great memories of you as my golf coach back in… well, sometime in the 80's. I have enjoyed talking to you at the country club whenever I am in town for the Rotary meetings! Thank you for being my friend and sponsoring my book!

Mary Lu Whaling… you and your family are the sweetest, most sophisticated, smart and loving folks around! Thank you for helping me with my book. You guys are the coolest cousins… see you at the Boxwoods at Christmas… well, hopefully sooner to deliver my book. Thank you for your donation!

Dear Anne and Dave… my loving aunt and uncle, who are so family oriented and loving! I hope I can come see you more, you are not that far away… we miss "A"… but she is always there guiding us… she is one of my favorite guardian angels…

Gene Bates, your trumbone is hypnotic… I want a personal serenade! Thank you for your awesome donation for my book… I love playing on the Big Band with you, you are so sweet and sexy!

Lisa Prilliman… you are like the 5th sister! Thank you so much for your donation! You have been in our family a very, very long time… and you better not go anywhere. No moving out west or anything like that… we love you!

Thank you ***Aunt Sandra***! You have always been that "cool" outlet for us. You know, aunts are supposedly cooler than moms, so thank you for living close by and for understanding me! I love your place and your big black lab… retriever!? Thank you for your donation for my book!

Thank you ***Daniel Donovan*** for being a loving sponsor and my long time friend! I love seeing you at our shows and hangin' out every couple of months. Thank you for being so cool and sweet!

Thank you ***Kerry Rhyne White*** for sponsoring my book! I love you and cannot wait til St. Gabriel visits you!

Thank you **Karen and Dan** for being a life sponsor of mine! I love you very much!

Thank You
To My Loving Family And Friends

Dear Dad,

You are the sweetest and kindest person on the planet! I love you. Thank you for helping me during this transition. Your gas cards and grocery vouchers have saved me. I am doing my very best right now, and I think you know that. Thank you for supporting me. Thank you for playing your beautiful sax with me when I sing. Thank you for sharing with me the gift of music, it renews the soul. Thank you for being my friend. I love you Papa Penn!

Dear Mom,

Thank you for the gift of life. You have been such a support for me during this transition and during the creation of this book. Thank you for being such an inspiration! Your job is so cool. You're so organized. I love to watch you strut your stuff at the rec center. You have literally written a grant for every cool thing in Madison. Madison wouldn't be Madison if it wasn't for you. Thank you for making our home so warm and perfect! It's like magic after you've touched just one room with your love and energy. Thank you for sharing your beautiful talents with me. I love to sing duets with you! Our arrangements are cool! Thanks for being my 'tanning' friend and shopping buddy. And thank you for your loving sponsorship. I love you.

Dear Vaughan,

Thank you for all of our wonderful memories! I love you... and love singing your beautiful music with you. You really are one of the best songwriters in history... I am not sure you know that. But you are! Your heart is so big, that you would fit the world in it if you could! Keep praying and singing and writing. I hope we can go out west together again one day. George is waiting.

Dear Elaine,

Thank you so much for being in our little world of Madison this year! I love having you home and watching you work. You are so motivated and focused. I love that. Thank you for motivating my focus for this book! Thank you for singing with us on the jazz bands… your songs are perfect! You are an excellent coach, I can't wait to come to one of your new programs. I'm so proud of you for making your life happen! I love you.

Dear Liz,

Thank you for being so good and grounded! 'A' trained you well. Your angelic perseverence in life gets you and keeps you in healthy and productive situations. You are such an inspiration! I am so proud of you for your second career! You have become who you are suppose to be and continuously attract more good to your life. I look forward to seeing those waterfalls with you soon and living in the same town one day… Madison or Williamsburg, either one. I love you!

Dear Deana,

Your creative soul is beautiful. You are so passionate and know how to live life fully every moment! Thank you for being in our lives over the past 18 years. Thank you for all the Christmas bows and amazing wooden bowls! Don't ever stop creating. Thank you for teaching me how to dance and perform back in the day… and thank you for being one of my favorite role models. Your dancers were so cute this year… we love having you close by! I love you… G-Anna

P.S. Thank you for your literary 'jumpstart' for this book! Divine!

Dear Tanya Kitty,

Thank you, Tanya Kitty, for being my very best friend and roommate! I was praying to God to bring me a friend I could play 'catch' with... I never imagined he would bring me you! Thank you for coming all the way down here into my life, you are an angel. You are so much fun, I love you.

Dear Tita,

Thank you Tita for clearing the way. And for being such a non-judging and loving little angel. Your excitement for life is precious. Do not ever stop dreaming and moving forward. Do you remember your mission statement for your life? Well, you have touched my life like a guiding light. Wow! Do you remember that day back in February when we thought maybe my poems would fit nicely into my letter? Well, I never imagined a real book would appear. Thank you for being, in essence, my life-coach over the past year… and my dear friend. Thank you for saving me over and over again! And for being my constant 'jumpstart.' You are fully living out your mission here on Earth. You can tell your angel you've touched my life, greatly. Thank you for blessing my life and blessing my journey. I love you Tita!

Dear Kerry,

Thank you Kerry for being my rock and best friend! Thank you so much for including me in your wedding day. You are such a confident inspiration. You know what you want, you set your mind to it and you go make it happen. Whether it's moving to L.A., getting a job or creating the life you want to live. Well, you are definitely becoming who you are suppose to become. Thank you for asking me, five years ago, how to pray. I have enjoyed watching you on your journey to Christ. I'm glad we've both found a church that we love! I love you… and thank you for being my favorite little peace of God. You are truly a gift to my journey.

Dear Karen, Dan and Ethan,

Thank you for being such great friends and role models. I love you and am so glad you found each other. Thank you for inviting me to St. Pius almost three years ago. Thank you, Gale, for being a part of my journey. And for creating such great miracles in your children and grandchild. You are a shining light.

Dear Tracy,

Tracy Earl Welliver, you are the 'heart' of this church. Thank you Tracy for your loving support and guidance; and knowing that 'I get it'… You definitely 'get it'. You are such an angelic and peaceful presence. Thank you for 'keeping' me on this journey. Thank you, Mariann, for being Tracy's other half. I truly believe that our loved ones help make us whole and make us who we are. Thank you for supporting Tracy while he carries out all his many missions!

Thank you Jodi for being my courage sponsor and for your inspiration and divine experience last year. Thank you, Jodi and Sanctuary House for the gift of courage!!

Thank you, Sue. Here is my thesis, my profession of faith… my final draft! You asked us to keep a journal in RCIA… and, well… here it is! Thank you for enduring all of my growing pains. I guess, sometimes, we just keep saving each other over and over again, kind of like Christ! Thank you for being my saving grace over the past two years. Thank you for being my friend and my official Catholic sponsor!

Thank you Donna for being such a great leader, speaker and teacher! Thank you for being a part of my journey! We love you! Thank you for being a part of the benefit concert last year! Can I join RCIA again? Maybe a third round? Thank you, Donna!

Thank you Hannah Hammer! You have inspired and guided me with your loving light and prayers! I love you! And thank you to all of St. Joseph's prayer group, you are such a support to this community! We love you!

Thank you, Hanna M. You are so strong and solid! I am so proud of you for all your many adventures out west. Thank you for the many vacations to the coast. Your creativity and art is so beautiful and calming! Iam so glad you can relate to the human condition. I pray to Goddess for you everyday to be happy and have peace.

Thank you also to your loving parents, Peggy and Jim for being our friends and fun neighbors... and for sharing their many many beautiful homes!

Thank you John Rodenbough for your guidance. I love you and your family. Y'all are precious gems along my journey. Thank you, John.

Thank you to all my Charlotte buddies, Kerry, Brad, Cindy and Lloyd, Katie, Stephanie, Tanya, Jennifer and Neal!

Thank you to all of my G.C. friends and roommates from many years ago. Thank you to Greensboro College for my wonderful education!

Thank you to all of my high school and childhood friends from Madison.

Thank you Ladonna.
Thank you Janet.
Thank you Michael P. for the fun job for me and Vaughanie on E.R.
Thank you Jeri Rowe for opening the portal
Thank you to the Key's for your guidance and inspiration!

Thank you Sylvia Via for being one of our Penn Pals!

Thank you to my early morning egg souffle buddies… thank you for the chats and support!

Thank you to Julie Hayes for your loving support.

Thank Alabaster Book Publishing. Thank you Dave for giving my book a home. And for the many hours at your computer, many hours. Thank you Dixie for your patience. I look forward to many more books to come.

Thank you to my pastor, Monsignor Marcaccio, for promising me that "one day, this will pass…" and for giving me the most precious gift of all… hope.

Thank you to all the visiting Priests at St. Pius X
Thank you Virginia
Thank you Bill & Shelley
Thank you Elly
Thank you M & M for reading my poems
Marilyn, I love your poetry book.
Thank you to the White's for being such a cool family for my best friend to be a part of now.
Thank you to my childhood Presbyterian minister
Thank you Rev. C. Howell
Thank you Tim, for your friendship and great sound.
Thank you all of our cool Madison friends
Thank you Greensboro College
Thank you to my freshman English professor for believing in me and teaching me how to write.

Thank you to all my angels and all the Saints that I am now calling on!!

Thank you to my wonderful family for giving me wings to fly and a safe ground to stand on. Thank you St. Pius. Thank you to all of our Madison friends for supporting our music! Thank you to my sister Elaine for your intellect and development expertise. Thank you mom & dad for the gift of music. Thank you Tita for clearing the way. Thank you Tracy. Thank you Deana for your literary excellence. Thank you Sue, thank you RCIA…

Thank you to all the deacons at St. Pius, Deacon Bill, Phil and Ron.

*Thank you to my sister Vaughan for your many, many prayers… I am truly guided by them and love you… and thank you for just being my sister! Written January 22nd, 2007 after many years of rough drafts! ***God Bless you all! ****

My Journey to Christ...

"It is not in any outward thing; such as forms, or ceremonies, even of the most excellent kind. No, the religion of Christ rises infinitely higher, and lies immensely deeper, than all these. These are good in their place; just as far as they are in fact subservient to true heart religion.

This faith is not in forms of worship, or rites and ceremonies, or outward actions. Neither is it right doctrine or intellectual belief.

No, it is a heart transformed by love, 'Thou shalt love the Lord thy God with all thy heart, and with all thy mind and with all thy soul, and with all thy strength… and thy neighbor as thy self.'"

John Wesley

Thank you St. Pius for putting ritual and ceremony to what I know in my heart.

Thank you St. Pius for putting words and intellect to what I know in my heart.

Thank you St. Pius for being that light to which I am drawn over, and over, and over again!

To the future…

....to stepping out
patiently,

in faith,

that is grounded

in hope, love and light!

Source Notes/Bibliography

GRP's Manual of Style

Pg. 5 Inspired by words spoken during the epiclesis at mass, summer 2005. Specific date unknown. Unpublished. Words appear to be a paraphrase of the following bible verse: *"In your prayers do not go babbling on like the heathen, who imagine that the more they say the more likely they are to be heard. Do not imitate them. Your father knows what your needs are before you ask him." Matthew 6:7-8 (New English Bible).*

Pg. 20 Mark Twain. Words seen on an inspirational chalk board in an ice cream shop in North Carolina. Secondary and original source of quote: Bartlett's Familiar Quotes, John Bartlett. 15th and 125th Anniversary Edition. Little, Brown and Company. Boston / Toronto. Pg. 624:15 *(ib.6)*. Pudd'nhead Wilson[1894]. Pudd'nhead Wilson's Calendar, Ch. I.

Pg. 23 Anonymous. (personal communication). Words spoken during conversation with author, fall 2005. Specific date unknown. Unpublished.

Pg. 37 Catechism of the Catholic Church. Second Edition: Revised *in accordance with the official Latin text promulgated by Pope John Paul II.* United States Catholic Conference, Inc. Libreria Editrice Vaticana. English Translation Copyright 1997,

USCC, Inc. http://www.usccb.org/catechism/text/pt1sect1.htm#chpt1. Paragraph 42. Footnote 16 is from *Liturgy of St. John Anaphora. This paragraph also takes you to 212,300,370.*

Pg. 37 Catechism of the Catholic Church. Second Edition: Revised *in accordance with the official Latin text promulgated by Pope John Paul II.* United States Catholic Conference, Inc. Libreria Editrice Vaticana. English Translation Copyright 1997, USCC, Inc. http://www.usccb.org/catechism/text/pt1sect1.htm#chpt1. Paragraph 40 (Man's Capacity for God) How can we speak of God?

Pg. 51 Sue Brusnahan. Friend and Catholic RCIA sponsor. (personal communication). Conversation held with author fall 2006. Exact date unknown. Unpublished.

Pg. 54 Anonymous. Words spoken at church sermon/homily. Summer 2005. Specific date unknown. Unpublished.

Pg.68 Anonymous. Conversation held in Greensboro, NC. (personal communication). Conversation held, summer 2007. Specific date unknown. Unpublished.

Pg. 76 Webster's Collegiate Dictionary. Second Edition. Depression.

Pg. 78 Barnes and Noble Concise Medical Dictionary. This edition is based on the New American Pocket Medical Dictionary, Second Edition by Nancy Roper © Churchill Livingstone 1988. Pg. 122. Depression.

Pg. 116 Fred Rogers. *Mister Rogers' Neighborhood* television show. Usage of quote inspired by Doneen Key's book, "Do You Want to Take Her Home?" Empire Publishing. Madison, NC. Pg. 3. Thank you Doneen for your inspiration. Original source unknown.

Pg. 125 Catechism of the Catholic Church. Second Edition: Revised *in accordance with the official Latin text promulgated by Pope John Paul II.* United States Catholic Conference, Inc. Libreria Editrice Vaticana. English Translation Copyright 1997, USCC, Inc. http://www.usccb.org/catechism/text/pt4sect1.htm. Paragraph 2563. What is Prayer? Prayer as covenant. It takes you to 2699 and 1696.

Pg. 129 Visiting Priest at St. Pius X Catholic Church in Greensboro, NC. Words spoken during the homily at mass, June 2005. Specific date unknown. Unpublished.

Pg. 206 Inspired by John Jackman's life of John Wesley script, "Wesley." Exact paraphrase of John Wesley's Sermon #7 by John P. Jackman. Pg. 130.

Based on orginal script by John Wells and Norman Stone. John P. Jackman. 2004. Registered, WGAW 1023624. Rev. 4.1 10/04/06. Secondary source and info on original source: http://new.gbgm-umc.org/umhistory/wesley/sermons/7/. Global Ministries United Methodist Church website. The Sermons of John Wesley. "The Way to the Kingdom." By: John Wesley, sermon 7. (Text from 1872 edition – Thomas Jackson, editor).

Pg. 219 Barnes and Noble Concise Medical Dictionary. This edition is based on the New American Pocket Medical Dictionary, Second edition by Nancy Roper © Churchill Livingstone, 1988. Pg. 90. Chronic Fatigue Syndrome.

Funny Words Reference Guide

Epiclesis – See Source Notes. Catholic term for calling down the Holy Spirit on to the gifts, *bread and wine*, during the communion prayers spoken by the Priest. It is that moment during the prayers that the Priest calls down the Holy Spirit onto the gifts asking the Holy Spirit to transform the bread and wine into the real body and blood of Christ. This epiclesis occurs in other sacraments as well.

Transubstantiation – This is the actual process or transformation during the Eucharist or Holy Communion where the bread and wine become the real body and blood of Christ. Epiclesis is the *time* when the transubstantiation occurs during the prayers during the Eucharist. In most Protestant churches, the bread and wine, or grape juice… are *symbolic* of the body and blood of Christ. But in the Catholic faith, because of its consecration, they believe the bread and wine actually *become* the real body and blood of Christ.

Vat of Holy Water – A small bowl, *not a large vessel or barrel*, holding holy water on each side of the entrance to St. Pius… *and many other Catholic churches.* Holy water is used before mass to remind us of our Baptism. Before I knew the reasoning behind the use of holy water… I just knew it felt healing and soothing, *emotionally and physically, to me! But, I am very guided by my heart and by feel. But, it does have an actual concrete meaning.* It is blessed by the Priest and used for sacramental purposes… as well as during special blessings performed by the Priest or Deacon. And, once again, it is a reminder of our Baptism, when we use it and make the sign of the cross!

St. Blaise - In the Catholic faith, he is referred to as the Patron Saint for the healing of throats. Pronuonced like, *St. Blaze.* For two years, I thought the Priest was saying St. Blaze or Blazen.

RCIA – Rite of Christian Initiation for Adults. It is the faith formation classes for adults who desire to be fully initiated into the Catholic faith. The actual faith formation process, the RCIA process, is a *rite* within itself.

Behind the Glass – In most Catholic Churches, they have what is called 'the cry room'. It is not the nursery, it is a room at the back or side of the church that parents can take their children and sit and still hear, see and participate in the mass. They can be in church with everyone else… just in a separate section. I like to call it my *cry room* or panic room… when I am in pain or not feeling well, I sit *behind the glass* so I can move around and go outside if I need to. Or, if mass is too emotionally intense for me that day, you can find me *behind the glass.*

Catechism of the Catholic Church – Big green book, or brown. A reference guide for the teachings of the Catholic Church, along with terminology and explanations of each teaching.

Sanctuary House – A psychosocial rehabilitation facility for adults recovering from severe mental illness. They provide social activities, a cantina, members cook meals and take classes and exercise together. It is part of a Clubhouse model program, which means the members are just that… members. They have an active role in the hiring of staff, in the planning and implementing of programs and of planning activities and managing the budget. It is amazing! Check out Sanctuary House… it is awesome! And please, if you like, make a contribution to their organization at www.sanctuaryhousegso.com

Have a Nice Day Project – That would be the beautiful groovy folk music of my dear friend, Tracy Earl Welliver. Check out his music at www.myspace.com/haveanicedaymusic

Purgatory – According to the Catholic faith, it is a place after death where some souls go to be cleansed and rehabilitated before entering

Heaven. It is not meant to have a negative connotation… *it simply is a place for further cleansing and rehabilitation for the soul, before entering Heaven.* Some souls are believed to go here and some are not in need of necessarily going here. I like to think of it like other faiths believe in reincarnation. From my understanding, some people believe that souls are reincarnated over and over again until they are good enough or evolved enough to go to Heaven. *To me, this reincarnation is sort of their purgatory.* *Pg. 92*

Grandma "A" - Our Guardian Angel!! My father's mother… the most precious and angelic person in almost all of the world!!

St. Francis – In the Catholic faith, St. Francis is the patron saint for animals. There is also another St. Francis. Look up the stories of St. Francis.

St. Gabriel – According to the Catholic faith, St. Gabriel is the patron saint for communications workers. He is also the angel who came to Mary and informed her she was to have a son, the son of God, and call him, Jesus. He would be born of a Virgin birth and be called our Savior. Angel Gabriel also came to Mary's cousin, Elizabeth, to inform her of having a son, John the Baptist. St. Gabriel is also the name of the Catholic Church in Charlotte, NC where my best friend, Kerry married her soulmate, Brad!

Myths and Truths of Mary – Mother Mary, mother of Jesus, our Lord, is highly revered in the Catholic Church. However, some Protestants and non-Catholics are extremely misinformed regarding Mary's role in the Catholic faith. Many believe that Catholics must go *through* Mary and the saints to reach God. They think of Catholics as *worshiping Mary.* Well, I guess you could say this is one of those *myths* of the Catholic Church. Mary is not adored, as Christ is… she is someone to which we are devoted.

Mary is highly revered, but not worshiped. She is merely an extra helper, an additional guide… and a great one at that; *since she has a special connection to our Lord, Jesus Christ.* Catholics do not have to go through Mary to pray to God, we merely pray to her asking her to pray for us. She is the ultimate intercessor.

It is sort of like this; *most people feel they have a guardian angel,* maybe a relative who has passed on, maybe a grandparent… who they feel compelled to pray to, *asking for guidance.* Well, in the Catholic faith, we pray to Mary and to the Saints… *and to our loved ones*, living and deceased, asking for their guidance and extra prayers!

Immaculate Conception – In the Catholic faith, this term refers to Mary's conception, when Mary was conceived. When she was conceived, by the Grace of God, she was born the most pure human of all man-kind. She was born free from Orginal Sin, to be able to be the perfect vessel for her son, Jesus Christ, to be born.

The Assumption – This is the day that Mary left this Earth and joined the Angels in Heaven. This day is very special in the Catholic Church and is considered a Holy Day of Obligation.

The Annunciation – This is the day when Angel Gabriel came to Mary and informed her she was to have a Son, and call him, Jesus. He was to be born of a Virgin Birth and be called, Savior.

The Rosary – The Rosary is a long beaded necklace with a cross at the bottom of it. The Rosary prayer is a meditative and reflective prayer. As you hold the Rosary, there is a prayer for each bead. The first prayer is the Our Father, *The Lord's Prayer…* then 10 Hail Mary's, and then the Glory Be. There are 5 decades of 10 beads. For each decade, there is a reflection on Christ's life. Look up the story and the prayers of the Rosary. They are so soothing! *The Rosary is not meant to be worn as jewelry, but, sometimes, I do carry it around my neck and heart! It just feels good and keeps me safe!*

Feast Days – Some saints have their own day of recognition, they call them feast days.

Chronic Fatigue Syndrome – "Characterized by various symptoms but usually including lymphadenopathy, low-grade fever, muscular or bone pain, impaired mental concentration, and recurrent fatigue. May continue for years; cause unknown." Barnes & Noble Concise Medical Dictionary. See Source Notes.

Fibromyalgia - A generalized pain and fatigue disorder characterized by muscular pain and chronic fatigue... also known as a soft-tissue disorder, causing pain in muscles, ligaments and tendons. It is similar to arthritis, but effects soft tissue and not joints.... luckily, it is not degenerative, but the symptoms of the inflammation and tightening of soft tissues is painful and exhausting. It is different in each suffering victim. It can be caused by any major stressor; an illnes, viral or bacterial, an injury, major change or mental stress.

Post Traumatic Stress Disorder – Traumatic event which causes victim to remain stuck in that response of helplessness.... Please see Suggested Reading on PTSD.

Suggested Reading

Catechism of the Catholic Church. Second Edition. Copyright 1997. See Source Notes for more informtion on this book and the website for this book.

Catholic & Christian *An Explanation of Commonly Misunderstood Catholic Beliefs* by Alan Schreck. 20th Anniversary Edition. Servant Books. Published by St. Anthony Messenger Press. Cincinnatti, Ohio.

Anatomy of the Spirit *The Seven Stages of Power and Healing* by Caroline Myss, PH.D. Three Rivers Press. New York. http://www.randomhouse.com/. Originally published by Harmony Books, a division of Crown Publishers, Inc. 1996. *This book acted as a bridge for me while I was in RCLA. It converted my universal spiritual language into a form which helped me relate to the traditional language of the Catholic Church. Thank you Carolyn Myss for speaking my language.*

Care of the Soul *A Guide for Cultivating Depth and Sacredness in Everyday Life* by Thomas Moore. HarperPerennial, *a division of* HarperCollins *Publishers.* Copyright © 1992. *I have not read this book in over five years. I just picked it up in August, 2007. Thank you Thomas Moore for reminding us to accommodate for all parts of ourselves.*

Waking the Tiger *Healing Trauma, An Innate Capacity to Transform Overwhelming Experiences* by Peter A. Levine with Ann Frederick. North Atlantic Books, Berkeley, California. Copyright © 1997. *Great book for anyone suffering from PTSD or Post Traumatic Stress Responses. I recommend this for anyone with chronic stress.*

John Wesley *Sermon 7, The Way to the Kingdom* . Please see Source Notes on Sermon 7.

Chicago Manual of Style Fifteenth Edition. The University of Chicago Press. Chicago and London. Published 2003. *Great reference guide for any writer.*

Epilogue

I hope you have enjoyed my journey through these hope-filled pages. I do not claim to be an expert on psychology, spirituality or religion. I just wanted to share my story of hope with you.

I am also not an expert on the Catholic Church. However, I do feel this church and parish have touched the very depths of my soul's journey. And I hope that all of you will, one day, find a place of peace and inspiration, a place of hope and faith, a place that touches and reaches the very depths of your soul.

As my friend, Tracy, so gracefully reminds us, *"having something to believe in, gives us wings to fly."* There are so many peaces of God to capture and share… so many in each moment. We just have to get out of our way… and out of God's way to be able to see what's right in front of us… and embrace them fully!

Thank you to my sister, Vaughanie, for praying that one day, "the Holy Spirit would touch my soul once again with the peace of God…"

The many, many, many
Peaces of God!
Thank you,and God Bless you all!

"It's peace he brings you… it's peace he lifts you with.
His love will keep you safe.
His love… his amazing grace."

Vaughan Penn

There are so many peaces of God
To embrace everyday…

Embrace them and share
Them as often
As you can…

With grace, dignity…
And joy!

G.Penn Aug. 10, 2007

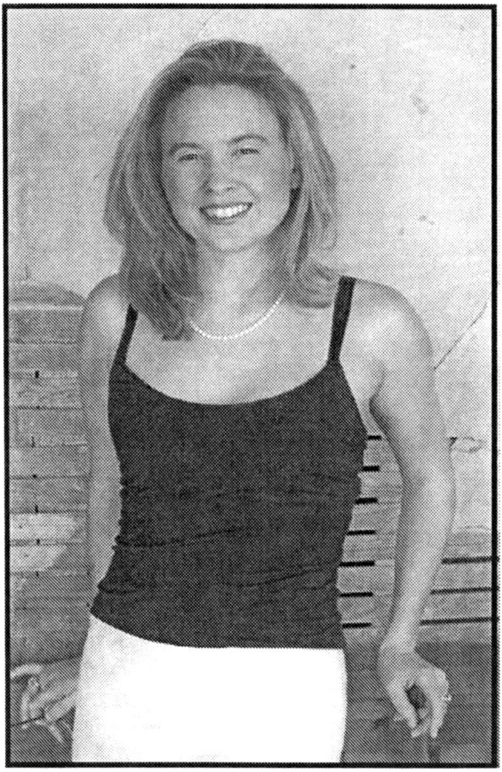

About The Author

Georgianna Penn grew up in Madison, N.C. She is a graduate of Greensboro College and has lived in Los Angeles, Virginia and throughout North Carolina. She has spent many years in sales, marketing and performing arts; and has recently rediscovered herself through art, poetry, creative writing… and her faith.

Thank you to
The Holy Spirit…For
The most precious gift
Of all…*hope.*

Printed in the United States
96882LV00001B/28-45/A